BEYOND DIAGNOSIS

BEYOND DIAGNOSIS

How To Develop Strong Relationships
Between Healthcare Providers
and Their Patients

PART OF THE
FOUNDATION OF HEALTHY
RELATIONSHIPS SERIES

R.E. GEFFNER, MD

Imar Publishing

ISBN (Paperback): 979-8-9952823-2-7
ISBN (eBook): 979-8-9952823-4-1
ISBN (Hardback): 979-8-9952823-3-4

Dedication

To the healers who stand at the threshold between uncertainty and hope—
This book is dedicated to you.

To the healthcare providers who carry the weight of life-altering decisions with steady hands and restless minds.
To the healthcare students who push through exhaustion in pursuit of mastery, fueled by a purpose greater than themselves.
To the healthcare provider assistants and nurse practitioners who bridge knowledge and compassion with quiet excellence.
To the nurses whose presence, more than any treatment, often becomes the true medicine.

To the managers who hold together the intricate systems that make healing possible.
To the caregivers, aides, and support staff whose work is too often unseen, yet deeply felt in every moment of dignity they preserve.

You are more than providers of care. You are witnesses to humanity at its most vulnerable and most real. You stand in rooms where fear, pain, hope, and love all coexist, often within the same breath. You navigate not only diagnoses and treatments, but emotions, families, and the fragile threads that connect one human being to another.

This book exists because of you and for you.

Because beyond every diagnosis is a person longing to be understood.
Because beyond every chart is a story waiting to be heard.
Because the greatest impact you will ever have is not only in what you treat, but in how you connect.

May these pages honor the strength you carry, the compassion you give, and the relationships you build, often in moments that matter most.

And may you always remember:
What you do saves lives.
How you do it transforms them.

Table of Contents

Dedication v
Preface xi
Introduction xv

Part I The Foundation of the Doctor–Patient Relationship 1

Chapter 1 The First Impression That Never Leaves 2
Chapter 2 Competence vs. Connection 19
Chapter 3 The Hidden Curriculum in Medicine 54
Chapter 4 Presence Over Perfection 58

Part II Communication That Builds or Breaks Trust 63

Chapter 5 The First Conversation 64
Chapter 6 Listening Beyond Symptoms 70
Chapter 7 Words That Land—and Words That Harm 75
Chapter 8 The 10-Minute Rule — Creating Meaningful Connections Even in Limited Time 98

Part III Navigating Difficult Clinical Scenarios 103

Chapter 9 Delivering Bad News 104
Chapter 10 When the Diagnosis Is Uncertain 127
Chapter 11 Managing Patient Anxiety and Fear 136
Chapter 12 The Angry or Distrustful Patient 158
Chapter 13 End-of-Life Conversations 175

Part IV The Healthcare Provider's Internal World 193

Chapter 14 Emotional Detachment vs. Emotional Control 194
Chapter 15 Burnout and Its Effect on Communication 201
Chapter 16 Time Pressure and Its Consequences 205
Chapter 17 Maintaining Humanity in a System That Demands Efficiency 210

Part V Teaching Relationship Skills in Medical Education **213**
Chapter 18 Why Relationship Training Must Start Early 214
Chapter 19 Role-Playing Real Scenarios 216
Chapter 20 Evaluating Communication Skills Objectively 236
Chapter 21 Feedback That Actually Improves Behavior 246
Chapter 22 Integrating Relationship Training into Clinical Rotations 260

Part VI A Practical Framework for Daily Practice **273**
Chapter 23 The 5-Step Interaction Model 274
Chapter 24 Micro-Skills That Make a Major Difference 283
Chapter 25 What Patients Remember Most 288
Chapter 26 Repairing a Damaged Interaction 292
Chapter 27 The 10-Second Orientation Rule 300
Chapter 28 The Waiting Room Problem 305
Chapter 29 Setting the Patient's Expectations — The Process Explained 312

Conclusion: The Healthcare Provider Patients Never Forget **317**

Acknowledgments 319
Appendix A 321
About the Author 363

Preface

Modern medicine is built on systems designed for movement: schedules to keep, metrics to meet, and a constant demand that must be sustained to keep the entire structure functioning. Efficiency is not optional; it is essential for access, coordination, and continuity of care. And yet, within this same system, healthcare providers are expected to deliver something that does not naturally conform to efficiency: human connection.

What is often missing is not awareness of its importance, but formal preparation for it. Many institutions of higher learning devote years to developing clinical knowledge, diagnostic accuracy, and technical skill, yet provide comparatively little structured education on how to build, maintain, and repair the healthcare provider–patient relationship. Communication is often treated as intuitive rather than teachable, and relational dynamics are absorbed informally rather than deliberately studied.

As a result, providers enter practice highly trained in disease management, but less prepared for the complexity of human interaction that defines daily care. The ability to navigate emotions, establish trust, manage expectations, and communicate with clarity under pressure is not consistently taught with the same rigor as physiology or pharmacology.

The consequence is not a lack of competence, but a gap in connection. In a system that prioritizes movement, the relational aspect of care can become underdeveloped—not because it is unimportant, but because it has not been given equal educational weight. And without that foundation, even the most advanced medical care can feel incomplete to the patient receiving it.

Acceptance into healthcare schools is one of the most defining moments in a person's life, not simply as an academic achievement but as entry into a profession entrusted with human life itself. It reflects a deep commitment to helping others—relieving suffering, treating illness, managing chronic disease, and increasingly preventing it to improve both longevity and quality of life. Yet, as medicine has advanced through technology, diagnostics, and scientific skill, an important imbalance has emerged. The human relationship between healthcare provider and patient—formed in the very first interaction—has not received equal emphasis. That initial connection determines whether a patient feels heard and respected, and, ultimately, whether they trust the care they receive. Without that trust, even the most advanced treatments can falter, be delayed, questioned, or not followed at all. While healthcare schools train providers in what to diagnose and how to treat, it has often neglected how to connect, communicate, and build trust, especially under emotional strain. These relational skills are not secondary; they are essential. The healthcare provider–patient relationship is not an addition to medicine—it is the foundation that allows medicine to work. For that reason, it should stand alongside clinical training as a central pillar of medical education, not at its periphery.

The Foundation That Is Often Overlooked

The Core Message

Patients do not need healthcare providers who feel nothing. They need healthcare providers who can feel—and still stay.

When individuals are accepted into healthcare schools, it is often one of the most meaningful and defining days of their lives. It represents more than academic achievement. It represents entry into a profession entrusted with human life itself. That acceptance is not simply an accomplishment. It is a profound privilege.

The vision that follows is equally powerful. The long path toward earning a degree in medicine, the discipline required, the responsibility assumed, and the eventual role of healthcare provider all carry a sense of purpose that is difficult to match. It is, in every sense, an extraordinary pursuit.

At the heart of that pursuit is a shared intention. Most healthcare students and healthcare providers begin with the same fundamental goal: to help people, to relieve suffering, to treat illness, to manage chronic disease, To reduce pain. And increasingly, to move beyond treatment into prevention. Modern medicine has evolved into a proactive force, aiming not only to cure disease but to extend life and improve its quality.

Where the Imbalance Begins

Yet within this progress, an imbalance has quietly developed. The advancement of medicine has been driven largely by:

- Technology
- Diagnostics
- Procedural skill
- Scientific knowledge

All of which are essential. All of which save lives. But in this evolution, one critical dimension has not received equal attention: The human relationship between healthcare provider and patient.

The Overlooked Truth

The first interaction between a doctor and a patient is not a minor moment; it is the foundation.

It determines:

- Whether the patient feels heard
- Whether they feel respected
- Whether they trust what follows

And that trust is not optional; it is central.

The Critical Point That I Am Making

Without trust and respect, even the most advanced medical care begins to weaken. Treatment may be:

- Delayed

- Questioned
- Incompletely followed
- Or entirely rejected

In other words, without the relationship, the medicine cannot fully work.

What Has Been Missing

Medical education has traditionally emphasized:

- What to diagnose
- How to treat
- When to intervene

But far less emphasis has been placed on:

- How to connect
- How to communicate
- How to build trust under pressure
- How to navigate emotional complexity

And yet, these are the very skills that determine whether a patient will engage in their own care.

The Conclusion

The relationship between providers and patients is not separate from medicine. It is what allows medicine to succeed. And for that reason, it should not be peripheral in medical education; it should be central to it.

This book addresses a quiet truth in medicine: patients rarely separate clinical skill from human connection. While technical excellence saves lives, it is the healthcare provider's presence that defines the experience of being cared for.

For decades, medical education has emphasized diagnosis, efficiency, and outcomes. Yet patients consistently describe their care in terms of how they were spoken to, whether they felt seen, and how difficult moments were handled.

As both a healthcare provider and a relationship expert. I have chosen to immerse myself in work that challenges a long-standing gap in training and offers a practical, teachable framework for restoring balance between competence and connection. This is not a critique of healthcare providers. It is an invitation to strengthen one of the most powerful tools in medicine: the doctor–patient relationship.

I will never forget the moment I chose to pursue a career in medicine. I was driven by both excitement and a deep sense of purpose, determined to become the best healthcare provider I could be. Even then, I understood that excellence in medicine would require more than technical skill. It would demand compassion, patience, and a genuine commitment to those who are suffering. I felt a strong and immediate empathy for individuals facing illness, and that awareness stayed with me throughout my journey.

Years of medical school followed, along with advanced training through multiple fellowships. During this long and demanding process, I refined not only my clinical abilities but also my capacity to connect with patients on a human level. I came to recognize that medicine is practiced not just through procedures and diagnoses, but through relationships.

Patients who entered the hospital or office were often stepping into the unknown. They carried fear, uncertainty, and quiet hope. They looked to their healthcare provider for reassurance, while bracing themselves for difficult news. In time, I learned that how we speak to patients is just as important as what we say. When we meet individuals at their level of understanding, with clarity and empathy, we give them more than information. We give them comfort, trust, and a sense of stability in an otherwise uncertain moment.

That realization shaped my approach to care. It became clear that the true art of medicine lies in the ability to combine knowledge with humanity, delivering not only answers, but also reassurance and dignity to every patient we serve.

As new healthcare professionals joined my practice, I made it a priority to share my approach to both teaching and patient care. I encouraged them to see each patient as an individual, not simply as a case. Every person brings a unique combination of personality, educational background, emotional state, and level of fear into the exam room. Because of this, communication cannot be one-size-fits-all. It must be adapted thoughtfully so that each patient can fully understand their condition and feel informed about their health.

I also reminded them of something equally important: authenticity matters. Titles and credentials may establish authority, but it is a genuine human connection that builds trust. I encouraged them to "let their guard down" and simply be themselves, because patients respond best to sincerity, not formality.

Finally, I emphasized that most health issues are not resolved in a single visit. Patients need to understand that diagnosis, treatment, and recovery are often part of a process that unfolds over time. Unless the visit is purely routine, clarity about this journey helps set realistic expectations and reduces anxiety. Our role is not only to treat but also to guide patients through that process with patience, honesty, and care.

I emphasized to my staff that mastering communication with patients is even more important than applying the technical skills they have worked so hard to learn. Clinical expertise is essential, but it is not what patients carry with them when they leave the room.

Patients may not remember every detail of what was explained to them, but they will always remember how their healthcare provider made them feel. That emotional experience becomes their lasting impression, shaping their trust, their confidence, and their willingness to follow through with care.

From the very first encounter, the tone of the relationship is established. The way a healthcare provider listens, speaks, and responds sets the foundation for all future interactions. When patients feel respected, understood, and genuinely cared for, communication becomes more effective, and the partnership between doctor and patient grows stronger.

Introduction

Why Relationships Are Not Optional in Medicine

There is a moment every patient remembers.

It is not always the diagnosis.

It is not always the treatment.

It is the interaction.

A tone.

A pause.

A sentence delivered too quickly—or with care.

Over years of practice, I observed something that is rarely taught but often felt: patients evaluate their healthcare providers not only by what they know, but by how they relate. In many cases, the relationship becomes the lens through which competence itself is judged.

Healthcare providers are deeply dedicated individuals. They work under pressure, carry enormous responsibility, and are trained to prioritize accuracy and efficiency. Yet within that training, one critical skill is often underdeveloped: how to be present with another human being in moments of fear, uncertainty, and grief.

This book is not about adding burdens to healthcare providers. It is about equipping them. It is about teaching:

- How to communicate when words matter most
- How to remain human in high-pressure environments
- How to deliver truth without removing hope
- How to recognize that *how* something is said can be as important as *what* is said

My goal is simple: to provide a framework that can be introduced early in medical training, so that future healthcare providers do not have to *learn this the hard way*, because in medicine, the healthcare provider-patient relationship is not a soft skill; it is a clinical skill.

Part I

The Foundation of the Doctor–Patient Relationship

Chapter 1	The First Impression That Never Leaves	2
Chapter 2	Competence vs. Connection	19
Chapter 3	The Hidden Curriculum in Medicine	54
Chapter 4	Presence Over Perfection	58

Chapter 1

The First Impression That Never Leaves

Why Initial Interactions shape Long-term Trust

Every patient you meet begins forming a judgment about you before you speak, before you examine them, and long before you offer a diagnosis. This judgment is not casual. It is not superficial. It is decisive. Within seconds, patients determine whether they trust you, whether they feel safe with you, and whether they believe you see them as a person or simply as a case. That decision quietly shapes everything that follows. It influences what they share, what they withhold, how they interpret your words, and whether they ultimately follow your care.

This is not a soft skill. This is not a secondary layer to clinical excellence. It is the foundation upon which all effective care is built.

Medical training emphasizes accuracy, efficiency, and decision-making under pressure. These are essential. But they do not operate in isolation. They are filtered through the patient's perception of you, and that perception is formed immediately. You are not first evaluated by what you know. You are first evaluated by how you show up. Before you say a single word, the patient has already begun forming a conclusion about you. Not an opinion. A conclusion.

It starts before you enter the room. They hear footsteps in the hallway. The rhythm matters. Fast, uneven, hurried steps signal something different from measured, steady movement. A rushed pace suggests pressure, distraction, or a lack of time. A controlled pace suggests intention and presence.

The door opens. Now the evaluation accelerates. Your attire is the first visible signal. Patients are not consciously analyzing it, but they are interpreting it instantly. A clean, well-fitted coat communicates order, discipline, and professionalism. Wrinkled clothing, stained fabric, or disorganization introduces doubt, even if subtle. Details matter more than healthcare providers are taught to believe. The way you present yourself answers an unspoken question: *Does this person take their role seriously enough to take me seriously?*

Your posture follows immediately. Do you enter upright, grounded, and aware of the space, or slightly hunched, already looking at a chart or screen? A downward gaze signals preoccupation. A direct, level posture signals readiness.

Your hands matter. Are they occupied with a device, typing, flipping through papers, or are they free, available, and open? Occupied hands often translate to divided attention.

Then comes eye contact. Not whether you make it, but **when** you make it. If your first visual connection is with a screen, a clipboard, or the floor, the patient registers that they are secondary. If your first connection is with the patient themselves, even briefly, it communicates priority.

And all of this occurs within seconds. Before your introduction. Before your first question. Before any clinical interaction begins.

Dialogue: The First Judgment Happens Before You Speak

(Patient sits alone in the exam room. They hear footsteps approaching—fast, uneven footsteps in the hallway.)

Patient (thinking):
That sounds rushed…

(Door opens quickly. Provider enters while looking at a tablet.)

Provider:
Hi, I'm Dr. Smith. What brings you in today? *(eyes still on screen)*

Patient:
Uh… I've been having some symptoms I'm worried about.

Provider:
Okay, go ahead. *(typing, minimal eye contact)*

Patient:
I'm not sure how serious it is… *(patient begins to hold back, uncertain)*

The same scenario unfolds again, but the provider enters differently this time, their measured, steady footsteps approaching the door.

Patient (thinking):
That sounds calm…

(Door opens at a natural pace. Provider pauses briefly, looks directly at the patient before stepping in.)

Provider:
Good morning, I'm Dr. Smith. *(makes eye contact, calm tone)*

Patient:
Hi…

Provider:
I'm glad you came in today. *(hands free, attentive posture)*

Patient:
Thank you…

Provider:
Before we get started, I want to make sure I'm fully focused on you. *(sets tone intentionally)*

Patient:
I appreciate that.

Provider:
What's been going on? Take your time. *(invites narrative)*

Patient:
I've been having symptoms, and I've been really worried about them.

(Patient leans in, more open)

Patient (thinking):
Okay… I feel comfortable talking to them.

Provider:
We'll go through this step by step and make sure you leave with clear answers. *(early leadership)*

Patient:
That makes me feel a lot better already.

Same provider. Same knowledge. But the moment of entry changes everything—long before a single clinical decision is made.

The Body Speaks Before You Do

Patients are highly attuned to nonverbal communication, especially in moments of vulnerability. They may not articulate what they are noticing, but they feel it with precision.

The angle of your body matters. Standing over a patient creates distance and hierarchy. Sitting, or at least lowering yourself to their level, reduces that distance and signals a willingness to engage.

The direction of your torso matters. If your body is angled toward the door, the patient senses that you are already leaving. If it is oriented toward them, they feel that you are staying.

Your movements matter. Quick, abrupt gestures can feel mechanical or impatient. Slower, deliberate movements suggest control and attentiveness. Even stillness matters. A provider who can pause, who is not constantly shifting or fidgeting, communicates a kind of quiet confidence that patients recognize immediately.

None of this is theatrical. It is perceptual. And patients are reading it continuously.

Dialogue: The Body Speaks Before You Do

(Provider enters and remains standing, slightly angled toward the door, tablet in hand.)

Provider:
What brings you in today? *(standing over patient; minimal eye contact)*

I've been having some symptoms that worry me…

Provider:
Okay. Go ahead. *(glances at the screen, shifts posture)*

Patient:
I'm not sure how serious it is.

(Provider taps on tablet, weight shifting, body still angled away)

Patient (thinking):
They seem distracted… maybe this isn't a big deal to them.

The same provider approaches differently this time. They step in, pause, meet the patient's eyes, and then sit at the patient's level, their body turned fully toward them.

Provider:
Hi, I'm Dr. Smith. *(calm tone, still posture)*

Patient:
Hi…

Provider:
I'm here with you—tell me what's been going on. *(Leans slightly forward, attentive)*

Patient:
I've been having symptoms that are really worrying me.

(Provider remains still, hands relaxed, no interruption)

Patient:
It's been getting worse, and I don't know what it means.

Provider:
I hear that it's been worsening, and that's understandably concerning. *(reflects, steady tone)*

Patient:
Yes, exactly.

(Provider nods slightly, maintains eye contact, no rushing)

Patient (thinking):
They're really listening…

Provider:
We'll go through this carefully, so you understand what's happening and what we'll do next. *(calm, grounded presence)*

Patient:
That makes me feel a lot better.

Even though the phrasing shifts from one scenario to the next, the real contrast isn't in the language — it's in the provider's presence.

The Voice That Sets the Tone

When you finally speak, your voice does not simply deliver words. It defines the emotional environment of the encounter. Tone, pace, and volume carry meaning before content is even processed. A rushed tone suggests urgency or a lack of time. A flat tone can feel detached or indifferent. A sharp tone may feel dismissive, even if unintended.

In contrast, a steady, measured tone communicates control. A slightly slowed pace signals that there is space for the patient. A warm but professional cadence communicates both competence and care. Even how you say the patient's name matters. If it is said quickly, as part of a routine, it feels procedural. If it is said with intention, it feels personal. This is not about being overly expressive. It is about being intentional.

Dialogue: The Voice That Sets the Tone

Provider:
Mr. Johnson, what seems to be the problem? *(fast, clipped tone)*

Patient:
I've been having some symptoms that worry me…

Provider:
Okay, go ahead. *(flat, rushed)*

Patient:
I'm not sure what's causing them.

Provider:
We'll check a few things. *(brief, detached)*

Patient:
…Alright.
They seem busy… I don't want to take too much time.

In another version of the encounter, the provider enters with a different voice, setting a different tone from the start.

Provider:
Mr. Johnson... *(slight pause, steady tone)*

Patient:
Yes?

Provider:
I'm glad you came in today. *(measured pace, warm but professional)*

Patient:
Thank you...

Provider:
Tell me what's been going on. Take your time. *(slightly slowed cadence)*

Patient:
I've been having symptoms that are worrying me.

Provider:
I hear that, and we'll go through this carefully together. *(steady, reassuring tone)*

Patient:
That makes me feel better already.

Provider:
I'm going to ask a few questions so I can understand this clearly. *(calm, controlled)*

Patient:
Okay.

Patient (thinking)**:**
They seem calm... like they know what they're doing.

Provider:
We'll make sure you leave here with clear answers and a plan. *(confident, grounded cadence)*

Patient:
I appreciate that.

The dialogue itself isn't the key difference here; it's the provider's voice, which can make the moment feel rushed or genuinely guided.

The Micro-Moments That Define You

There are specific micro-moments in the first 10 to 20 seconds that disproportionately shape the patient's perception:

- Whether you knock before entering
- Whether you pause after entering or move immediately into tasks
- Whether you introduce yourself clearly or assume your role is understood
- Whether you acknowledge the patient before interacting with the environment
- Whether you sit down or remain standing

Each of these moments answers a silent question the patient is asking: *Am I being treated as a person or processed as a task?*

Dialogue: The Micro-Moments That Define You

(No knock. Door opens quickly. Provider walks in while looking at a chart.)

Provider:
Hi. What brings you in? *(no introduction, immediate task focus)*

Patient:
Uh… I've been having some symptoms.

(Provider moves to computer, begins typing without sitting)

Provider:
Go ahead. *(attention split)*

Patient:
I'm not sure how serious it is…

(No pause, no acknowledgment)

Patient (thinking):
This feels rushed… like I'm just another appointment.

The same encounter unfolds again, but the micro-moments shift, creating a different experience.

(Knock on the door.)

Provider:
May I come in? *(respect for space)*

Patient:
Yes.

(Provider enters, pauses briefly, makes eye contact before doing anything else.)

Provider:
Good morning, I'm Dr. Smith. *(clear introduction)*

Patient:
Hi…

Provider:
It's nice to meet you. *(acknowledges person first)*
(Provider sits down at patient's level, body oriented toward them.)

Patient:
Nice to meet you too.

Provider:
Before I look at anything else, I want to hear what's been going on from your perspective. *(patient prioritized)*

Patient:
I've been having symptoms that worry me.

(Provider remains still, attentive, not rushing onto the computer.)

Patient (thinking):
Okay… they're actually here with me.

Provider:
We'll go through this step by step so you feel clear about what's happening. *(early leadership)*

Patient:
That already makes me feel better.

The provider hasn't changed, nor has their clinical knowledge. What shifts is the first twenty seconds. And in that shift, the patient moves from questioning, Am I being processed? to feeling, I matter here.

The Patient's Internal Calculation

While all of this is happening, the patient is performing a rapid internal calculation:

Is this provider paying attention to me?

Do they seem rushed?

Do they seem confident?

Do they seem to care?

Can I trust what they are about to tell me?

This calculation is not logical in the traditional sense. It is emotional, intuitive, and immediate. And once it is made, it becomes the lens through which everything else is interpreted. If the answer leans toward trust, the patient opens. If it leans toward doubt, the patient guards.

Dialogue: The Patient's Internal Calculation

(Provider enters quickly, glancing at the computer before the patient.)

Provider:
Hi, what's going on? *(rushed tone)*

Patient:
I've been having some symptoms that concern me…

Provider:
Okay, go ahead. *(typing, minimal eye contact)*

Patient:
I'm not sure what it means.

(Provider nods briefly but continues typing)

Patient (thinking):
Are they really paying attention? They seem rushed… Do they even see me?

Provider:
We'll run some tests. *(brief, no explanation)*

Patient:
Okay…

Patient (thinking):
I don't feel very confident… I'm not sure I trust this…

(Patient becomes more reserved, shares less)

The scenario is the same, but the signals shift as the encounter begins again.

(Provider enters calmly, makes eye contact first, sits down.)

Provider:
Hi, I'm Dr. Smith. I'm glad you came in. *(steady tone)*

Patient:
Thank you…

Provider:
I want to make sure I understand what's been going on—tell me in your own words.
(attentive, present)

Patient:
I've been having symptoms that are worrying me.

(Provider listens without interruption, slight nod, no rushing)

Patient (thinking):
They're paying attention… They seem calm… They care…

Provider:
We'll go through this carefully, and I'll make sure you have a clear plan moving forward. *(confidence + direction)*

Patient:
That helps a lot.

Patient (thinking):
I feel like I can trust this.

(Patient opens up, shares more, engages more fully)

The clinical scenario doesn't change, yet the patient's internal calculation does. That quiet shift determines the course of the entire encounter.

Why This Happens So Quickly

Patients do not have the luxury of time to evaluate you analytically. They rely on rapid pattern recognition, drawing from past experiences, fears, and expectations.

In a vulnerable state, the brain prioritizes one question above all: *"Am I safe here?"* Safety, in this context, is not just physical. It is psychological. It is the sense that the person in front of them is competent, attentive, and willing to engage with them as a human being. And that sense is formed almost instantly.

Dialogue: Why This Happens So Quickly

(Patient sits alone, visibly anxious, waiting. Door opens.)

Provider:
Hi, what's going on today? *(quick, neutral tone, minimal eye contact)*

Patient:
I've been having symptoms that really worry me…

Provider:
Okay, tell me. *(standing, glancing at screen)*

Patient:
I'm not sure what it means.

(Provider types while patient speaks)

Patient (thinking):
Something feels off… They seem distracted… "Am I safe here?

Provider:
We'll run some tests and see. *(brief, no reassurance or structure)*

Patient:
Okay…

Patient (thinking):
I don't feel very confident… I'm not sure I trust this…

(Patient becomes guarded, shares less)

The encounter repeats, yet the signals change, setting a different tone from the start.

(Door opens at a measured pace. Provider pauses, makes eye contact before speaking.)

Provider:
Hi, I'm Dr. Smith. *(steady tone)*

Patient:
Hi…

Provider:
I'm glad you came in today. *(calm, present)*

Patient:
Thank you…

Provider:
Before we begin, I want you to know we'll take this step by step so you feel clear and supported. *(sets psychological safety)*

Patient:
That helps already.

Provider:
Tell me what's been going on, in your own words. *(invites narrative)*

Patient:
I've been having symptoms that really worry me.

(Provider listens without interruption, still posture)

Patient (thinking):
They're focused... They seem steady... I think I'm okay here.

Provider:
We'll work through this together and make sure you have clear answers and a plan. *(confidence + direction)*

Patient:
I feel a lot better hearing that.

The scenario remains the same, but the patient's internal calculation shifts. Within seconds, they're assessing one essential question—*Am I safe here*—and that assessment determines the course of the encounter.

The Irreversibility of the First Impression

Once this initial impression is formed, it does not disappear. It anchors the interaction. If the first impression is strong, it creates resilience. Small missteps are forgiven. Communication flows more easily. Trust deepens. If the first impression is weak, it creates resistance. Even correct information may be questioned. Even appropriate care may feel insufficient.

This is why first impressions are not just important. They are structurally influential. They shape the trajectory of the entire relationship.

Dialogue: The Irreversibility of the First Impression

The first scenario opens with a weak initial impression that shapes the rest of the interaction.

(Door opens quickly. Provider enters without knocking, glancing at computer.)

Provider:
Hi, what's going on? *(rushed, minimal presence)*

Patient:
I've been having symptoms that worry me...

Provider:
Okay, tell me. *(typing, not fully engaged)*

Patient:
I'm not sure what it means.

(Patient begins to feel uncertain early)

Provider:
Your results look reassuring. There's nothing serious. *(correct information)*

Patient:
Are you sure?

Provider:
Yes, this is common. *(technically accurate)*

Patient:
I still feel uneasy...

(Despite receiving appropriate care, doubt lingers because the first impression is weak.)

Patient (thinking):
"I don't know... something just doesn't feel right."

In the second scenario, the encounter begins with a strong initial impression.

(Knock. Door opens calmly. Provider makes eye contact before speaking.)

Provider:
Hi, I'm Dr. Smith. I'm glad you came in. *(present, steady)*

Patient:
Thank you...

Provider:
We'll go through everything carefully, so you feel clear about what's happening. *(early leadership)*

Patient:
That helps already.

(Patient feels grounded from the start)

Provider:
Your results look reassuring. There's nothing suggesting a serious issue. *(same clinical information)*

Patient:
That's good to hear.

Provider:
I'll explain what we're seeing and why we're confident about that. *(clarity + guidance)*

Patient:
I appreciate that.

(A small change in presence creates a very different reception.)

Patient (thinking):
I trust what they're telling me.

In the first scenario, the patient pushes back against information that is clinically sound. In the second, that same information lands as steadying and reassuring. The divergence is created in the first moments — and it shapes everything that follows.

The Responsibility You Carry

It is easy, especially in a busy clinical environment, to view each encounter as routine. For the patient, it is not. They may have been thinking about this visit for days. They may be carrying fear they have not voiced. They may be deciding, in real time, whether they can trust you with information that matters. And all of that is influenced before you ask your first question.

Dialogue: The Responsibility You Carry

(Patient sits quietly, hands clasped, visibly anxious before the provider enters. Door opens quickly. Provider walks in while reviewing notes.)

Provider:
Hi, what brings you in today? *(routine, distracted)*

Patient:
I've been… thinking about this visit a lot.

Provider:
Okay, go ahead. *(typing, minimal eye contact)*

Patient:
I wasn't even sure if I should say everything…

(Patient hesitates, holds back)

Patient (thinking):
Maybe it's not important… Maybe I shouldn't mention it…

In the second scenario, the provider begins with a different awareness of their responsibility.

(Knock. Door opens calmly. Provider pauses, makes eye contact before speaking.)

Provider:
Hi, I'm Dr. Smith. I'm glad you came in. *(present, intentional)*

Patient:
Thank you…

Provider:
Before we start, I want you to know this is your time, and I'm here to listen carefully. *(creates safety)*

Patient:
That means a lot.

Provider:
Take your time—what's been on your mind? *(Invites openness)*

Patient:
I've been worried about something, but I wasn't sure if I should say it…

Provider:
If it matters to you, it matters here. *(validates importance)*

Patient:
I've been having symptoms I'm scared might be serious.

(Patient leans forward, more open)

Patient (thinking):
Okay… I can say this here.

Provider:
I'm really glad you shared that. We'll go through it carefully, so you feel clear and supported.
(guidance + reassurance)

Patient:
I feel better already.

The patient is the same, and so is the concern. In one scenario, it remains unspoken. In the other, it comes forward — made possible by a provider who recognizes the responsibility of those first moments.

A Standard Worth Holding

To practice medicine at the highest level requires more than diagnostic accuracy. It requires awareness of how you are perceived in the first moments of contact. Not as performance. Not as manipulation. But as a deliberate commitment to presence, respect, and clarity. Because before patients evaluate what you know, they evaluate who you are in the room. And that evaluation begins the moment you enter.

Dialogue: A Standard Worth Holding

(Patient sits waiting, anxious, thinking about the visit. Door opens abruptly. Provider walks in while glancing at notes.)

Provider:
Hi, what's going on today? *(routine, distracted)*

Patient:
I've been worried about something…

Provider:
Okay, go ahead. *(standing, divided attention)*

Patient:
I'm not sure how serious it is.

(Patient hesitates, senses lack of presence)

Patient (thinking):
I don't feel fully comfortable…

In the second scenario, the situation and the provider remain the same—but the standard they bring to the moment is different.

(Knock. Door opens calmly. Provider pauses, makes eye contact before speaking.)

Provider:
Hi, I'm Dr. Smith. It's good to meet you. *(intentional presence)*

Patient:
Hi…

Provider:
I'm glad you came in today. *(respect + acknowledgment)*

(Provider sits, body oriented toward patient, hands relaxed.)

Provider:
Before we begin, I want you to know I'm here to listen carefully and make sure you leave with clear answers. *(clarity + commitment)*

Patient:
That makes me feel better already.

Provider:
Take your time—what's been on your mind? *(invites openness)*

Patient:
I've been worried about something and didn't know who to talk to.

Provider:
I'm really glad you're sharing it here. *(validation)*

Patient:
Thank you…

(Patient leans in, more open)

Patient (thinking):
Okay… I feel like I can trust this.

Provider:
We'll go through this step by step so you feel clear and supported. *(leadership + presence)*

Patient:
I appreciate that.

The clinical encounter doesn't change, but the opening moments do. One version unfolds like a routine task; the other carries a sense of intention. In that contrast, the patient forms more than an impression of your knowledge—they form an impression of you.

Chapter 2

Competence vs. Connection

Why Patients Judge Both — And Often Merge Them

A provider can be clinically exceptional and still fail a patient. Not because the diagnosis was wrong. Not because the treatment was inappropriate. But because the patient did not feel understood, seen, or guided with care.

In medicine, competence and connection are often taught as separate domains. One belongs to science. The other to communication. One is measurable. The other is assumed. But in the patient's experience, they are not separate at all. They are fused. And once fused, they become indistinguishable.

Dialogue: Competence vs. Connection

Provider:
Your imaging shows a herniated disc at L4-L5. The treatment plan is anti-inflammatories and physical therapy. *(competent, but clinical)*

Patient:
Okay... is that serious?

Provider:
It's a common condition. We see this frequently. *(competent, but distancing)*

Patient:
It doesn't feel common to me... it's affecting everything I do.

Provider:
The prognosis is generally good with adherence to therapy. *(Technically correct, emotionally neutral)*

Patient:
I'm worried I won't be able to work.

Provider:
Most patients improve. *(minimizes individual concern)*

Patient:
...Alright.

(Patient leaves uncertain, unconvinced despite correct care)

In the second scenario, nothing about the diagnosis changes — only the standard the provider brings to the moment.

Provider:
Your imaging does show a disc issue in your lower back, which helps explain the pain you've been feeling. *(competence + clarity)*

Patient:
That makes sense...

Provider:
I also want to understand how this is affecting your day-to-day life. *(connection begins)*

Patient:
I can barely get through work, and that scares me.

Provider:
That's important for me to hear. Your ability to function matters just as much as the scan results. *(connection reinforces competence)*

Patient:
Thank you...

Provider:
The good news is we have effective ways to treat this, like medication and physical therapy. *(competence framed with reassurance)*

Patient:
Will I be able to work again normally?

Provider:
Most people do improve, but we'll tailor this to you and adjust based on how your body responds. *(balanced competence + individualized care)*

Patient:
That makes me feel more confident.

Provider:
We'll go through this step by step, and I'll make sure you're supported along the way. *(connection solidifies trust)*

Patient:
I feel a lot better hearing it explained this way.

Provider:
My goal isn't just to treat the condition, but to help you get back to your life. *(competence + purpose aligned)*

Patient:
Now I feel like you really understand what I'm going through.

The Patient's Single Question

Patients do not evaluate you in categories. They do not sit in the exam room thinking: "This provider is highly competent but emotionally distant." Instead, their mind simplifies everything into one overarching question: *"Can I trust this person with my health—and by extension, my life?"* That question absorbs everything you do. Your explanation of the diagnosis. Your eye contact. Your tone. Your ability to listen. Your confidence. Your presence. It all blends into a single perception.

When connection is absent, competence becomes the patient's only reference point, and the relationship is evaluated entirely through that limited frame. The problem is that the patient cannot judge competence as clearly as he can the connection because the patient has not been able to fully evaluate the provider's skill.

Providers are judged on their level of clinical competence, not their strength through their ability to connect.

Let us emphasize that the patient is there to seek the comfort of connection, but primarily there seeking clinical evaluation. They come because something is wrong, or might be wrong, and they need clarity, direction, and protection, but the connection is the first to be judged.

At a very basic level, the patient is asking:

- *What is happening to me?*
- *How serious is it?*
- *What are we going to do about it?*

These are not abstract questions. They are tied to fear, uncertainty, and sometimes survival.

Now imagine those questions are met with warmth, attentiveness, and kindness... but without clear, confident answers. The patient may feel liked. They may feel heard. But they do not feel anchored. And without that anchor, the connection begins to feel incomplete.

Dialogue: The Patient's Single Question

Provider:
So, tell me what's been going on. *(warm, attentive)*

Patient:
I've been having these symptoms, and I'm really worried.

Provider:
I can see this has been stressful for you. *(connection)*

Patient:
It has… I just don't know what's happening.

Provider:
You're not alone—we'll get through this together. *(connection, but vague)*

Patient:
Okay… but what do you think it is?

Provider:
It could be a number of things. *(unclear, lacks direction)*

Patient:
Is it serious?

Provider:
Try not to worry too much right now. *(reassuring, but unanchored)*

Patient:
I'm still worried…

(Patient feels heard—but uncertain, ungrounded)

The scenario repeats from the same point, but now the provider responds with a clearer, more grounded standard.

Provider:
I can see how much this has been weighing on you, and I'm really glad you came in. *(connection)*

Patient:
Thank you…

Provider:
Based on what you've told me so far, there are a few possible causes, and most are manageable. *(competence begins to anchor)*

Patient:
That's a relief…

Provider:
The next step is to run a few tests so we can be certain about what's going on. *(clear direction)*

Patient:
Okay, that makes sense.

Patient:
How serious do you think this is?

Provider:
Right now, nothing suggests an immediate danger, but it's important that we evaluate it carefully. *(balanced clarity)*

Patient:
I feel better hearing that.

Patient:
And what are we going to do about it?

Provider:
We'll move step by step—first getting clear answers, then deciding on the best treatment based on what we find. *(structure + plan)*

Patient:
That helps me feel more in control.

Provider:
My goal is not only to understand what's happening, but to guide you through it so you don't feel alone in the process. *(connection + competence fused)*

Patient:
Now I feel like I can trust this.

Why Warmth Alone Is Not Enough

Human beings are wired to seek both emotional safety and direction when they feel vulnerable. Connection provides emotional safety; competence provides direction. When connection is present, but competence feels uncertain, the brain begins to register a subtle mismatch: *"This person cares about me… but can they actually help me?"* That question creates tension. And in that tension, the warmth starts to lose its grounding. It begins to feel less like reassurance and more like compensation. Not intentionally. Not consciously. But perceptually.

Provider:
I'm really glad you came in today. I can tell this has been hard for you. *(warmth)*

Patient:
It has… I've been really worried.

Provider:
That makes complete sense. Anyone would feel that way. *(emotional validation)*

Patient:
Thank you…

Provider:
You're not alone in this. I'm here for you. *(supportive, but vague)*

Patient:
I appreciate that... but what do you think is going on?

Provider:
It's hard to say right now. *(uncertain, no direction)*

Patient:
Is it something serious?

Provider:
Try not to worry too much. We'll figure it out. *(reassurance without clarity)*

Patient:
I'm still worried...

(Patient feels cared for—but not guided)

The scenario continues from the same point, but now the provider responds with a clearer, more grounded standard.

Provider:
I can see how much this has been weighing on you, and I'm really glad you came in. *(warmth)*

Patient:
Thank you...

Provider:
Based on what you've told me and what I'm seeing, there are a few likely possibilities, and most are treatable. *(competence introduced)*

Patient:
That's reassuring...

Provider:
I'd like to run some tests so we can be precise about what's going on. *(clear direction)*

Patient:
Okay, that helps.

Patient:
So, you have an idea of what this could be?

Provider:
Yes, and we'll narrow it down step by step, so nothing is missed. *(confidence + process)*

Patient:
I feel better hearing that.

Provider:
I want you to feel supported, but also confident that we have a clear plan moving forward.
(connection + competence aligned)

Patient:
That makes a big difference.

Provider:
We'll go through this together, and I'll make sure you understand each step along the way.
(Guidance + presence)

Patient:
Now I feel like I'm in the right place.

How Patients Detect "Uncertain Competence"

Patients are not trained clinicians, but they are highly sensitive to certain signals that suggest uncertainty:

- Vague explanations without structure
- Hesitation that lacks clarity ("It could be a few things… we'll see…")
- Overuse of generalities instead of specifics
- Lack of a clear next step
- Inconsistent or shifting recommendations
- Avoidance of direct answers

Even subtle cues matter. If a provider cannot clearly explain what they are thinking, patients often assume the provider is not sure what they are doing. And once that perception forms, it affects how everything else is interpreted.

Dialogue: How Patients Detect "Uncertain Competence"

Provider:
It could be a few things… we'll just have to see. *(vague, no structure)*

Patient:
What kinds of things?

Provider:
Just different possibilities. *(general, non-specific)*

Patient:
That doesn't really help me understand…

Provider:
Let's just wait and see how it goes. *(no clear plan)*

Patient:
So… we're not doing anything?

Provider:
Not right now. *(lacks direction)*

Patient:
That makes me nervous.

(Patient begins to question provider's competence, despite no actual clinical error)

The scenario continues from the same point, but now the provider responds with a more structured, grounded standard.

Provider:
Based on what you've told me, there are a few specific possibilities I'm considering. *(structured thinking)*

Patient:
Okay, that helps.

Provider:
The most likely causes are A, B, and C, and each has a different way we evaluate it. *(organized clarity)*

Patient:
That makes more sense.

Patient:
So, what happens next?

Provider:
The next step is to run targeted tests to narrow this down. *(clear direction)*

Patient:
Good, I was hoping for a plan.

Patient:
Is this something serious?

Provider:
Right now, nothing suggests an urgent issue, but it's important we evaluate it carefully. *(balanced clarity)*

Patient:
That reassures me.

Provider:
Once we have the results, we'll review them together and decide on the best course of action. *(defined process)*

Patient:
I feel a lot more confident now.

Provider:
If anything changes before then, I want you to reach out so we can adjust quickly. *(continuity + control)*

Patient:
Thank you... now I feel like there's a clear path forward.

The Emotional Reversal

Here is where the phrase becomes most important. When competence feels uncertain, the patient begins to reinterpret the connection. What initially felt like kindness may now feel like:

- Softness instead of strength
- Politeness instead of leadership
- Comfort instead of guidance
- Incompetence disguised by a warm connection

The patient may not say this out loud, but internally, the shift happens: *"They're very nice... but I'm not confident in them."* And once that thought appears, the emotional weight of the connection weakens. That is what is meant by "hollow." Not fake. Not insincere. But lacking the substance needed to support trust fully.

Dialogue: The Emotional Reversal

Provider:
I'm really glad you came in. I can see how difficult this has been for you. *(warmth)*

Patient:
It has... I've been really worried.

Provider:
That makes complete sense. I'm here with you through this. *(connection)*

Patient:
Thank you...

Patient:
So, what do you think is going on?

Provider:
It could be a few things... it's hard to say right now. *(uncertain competence)*

Patient:
Like what?

Provider:
We'll just have to wait and see how things develop. *(no direction)*

Patient:
That's... not very reassuring.

(Internal shift begins)

Provider:
But you're not alone. I'll be here for you. *(continued warmth)*

Patient:
I appreciate that...

(Patient thinking:
"They're very nice... but I'm not confident in them.")

Patient:
Is there anything we should be doing right now?

Provider:
Let's not rush into anything. *(softness without leadership)*

Patient:
I feel like we should have a plan...

(Connection begins to feel hollow, not because it's insincere—but because it lacks direction)

In the second scenario, nothing about the patient's worry changes — only the standard the provider brings to the moment.

Provider:
I want to support you through this, and I also want to be clear about how we move forward. *(connection + leadership)*

Patient:
Okay...

Provider:
Based on what I'm seeing, there are a few likely causes, and here's how we'll sort them out. *(restores competence)*

Patient:
That's what I needed to hear.

Provider:
The next step is specific testing so we can get clear answers, and I'll guide you through each part. *(structure + direction)*

Patient:
I feel more confident now.

Provider:
My goal is not just to be here with you, but to lead you through this in a way that feels clear and steady. *(connection anchored in competence)*

Patient:
Now it doesn't just feel supportive... it feels solid.

The Role of Leadership

Patients are not just looking for a kind person. They are looking for someone who can lead them through uncertainty. Leadership in medicine is not dominance or authority in the traditional sense. It is clarity, structure, and direction delivered in a way that the patient can understand and accept. When that leadership is present:

- Connection deepens.
- Trust stabilizes.
- Anxiety decreases.

When that leadership is absent:

- Connection becomes fragile.
- Trust becomes conditional.
- Anxiety persists.

Dialogue: The Role of Leadership

Patient:
I've been feeling worse, and I don't know what's happening.

Provider:
I'm really sorry you're going through this. *(warmth)*

Patient:
Thank you... but what should we do?

Provider:
We'll just take it one day at a time. *(lacks direction)*

Patient:
That doesn't really give me a plan...

Provider:
Try not to worry too much. *(reassurance without structure)*

Patient:
I'm still worried.

(Connection present, but no leadership—anxiety remains)

The scenario continues from the same point, but now the provider responds with a clearer, more grounded standard.

Provider:
I can see how concerning this is, and I want to help guide you through it clearly. *(warmth + leadership)*

Patient:
Okay…

Provider:
Based on what you've told me, there are a few likely causes we need to evaluate. *(clarity)*

Patient:
That helps already.

Provider:
The first step is to run specific tests so we can narrow this down. *(direction)*

Patient:
Good, I needed to know what comes next.

Patient:
Is this something serious?

Provider:
Right now, nothing suggests an immediate danger, but it's important we address it carefully. *(balanced confidence)*

Patient:
That reassures me.

Provider:
After the tests, we'll review the results together and decide on the best course of action. *(structure)*

Patient:
I feel more in control now.

Provider:
My role is not just to support you, but to lead you through this in a way that feels clear and steady. *(leadership defined)*

Patient:
That's exactly what I need.

Provider:
You won't have to figure this out alone—we'll move forward step by step. *(connection anchored in leadership)*

Patient:
I feel much less anxious now.

A Simple Contrast

Consider these two interactions:

Provider A (warm, attentive, empathetic,):
Let's just monitor this and see what happens… it's probably nothing… we'll figure it out.

Provider B (also warm and attentive):
Based on what you've told me and what I'm seeing, here are the two most likely possibilities. The good news is that neither appears immediately dangerous. The next step is this test, and here's why it matters.

Both are kind. But only one provides structure, clarity, and direction. The second provider's connection feels solid because it is supported by competence that is clearly communicated.

The Integration That Must Happen

The goal is not to choose between being compassionate and being competent.
It is to ensure that your compassion is *backed by clarity*, and your competence is *delivered with humanity*.
When both are present:

- The patient feels cared for.
- The patient feels guided.
- The patient feels safe.

When one is missing, the experience becomes incomplete.

Dialogue: The Integration That Must Happen

Patient:
I've been really anxious about these symptoms.

Provider:
I'm sorry you're going through this. *(compassion only)*

Patient:
Thank you… do you know what's causing it?

Provider:
It's hard to say right now. *(lacks clarity)*

Patient:
So… what should I do?

Provider:
Just try to stay calm. *(compassion without direction)*

Patient:
I still feel unsure…

(Patient feels cared for, but not guided)

The scenario continues from the same point, but now the provider responds with a clearer, more grounded standard.

Provider:
I can see how much this has been weighing on you. *(compassion)*

Patient:
It really has.

Provider:
Based on what you've told me, there are a few likely causes we should look into. *(competence)*

Patient:
Okay…

Provider:
The next step is to run some specific tests so we can get clear answers. *(direction)*

Patient:
That helps me understand what's happening.

Patient:
Is this something serious?

Provider:
Right now, nothing suggests an immediate danger, but it's important we evaluate it carefully. *(balanced clarity)*

Patient:
That reassures me.

Provider:
We'll go through this step by step, and I'll make sure you understand each part along the way. *(guidance + presence)*

Patient:
I feel more at ease now.

Provider:
My goal is not just to care for you, but to guide you with clear, thoughtful decisions.
(integration defined)

Patient:
That makes me feel both supported and confident.

Provider:
When we combine both, you don't just feel heard—you feel safe moving forward.
(Integration complete)

Patient:
That's exactly how I feel right now.

The Deeper Truth

Patients do not separate who you are from what you know. If they feel unsure about your competence, it changes how they experience your presence. And if they feel unsure about your presence, it changes how they interpret your competence. This is why the integration matters so deeply.

The Highlight

Connection without competence can comfort a patient for a moment. But competence, clearly communicated and delivered with connection, can steady a patient through uncertainty. And that is what they are truly seeking. If competence appears uncertain, connection feels hollow. To the patient, these are not two qualities. They are one experience.

Dialogue: When Connection Feels Hollow Without Competence

Provider:
I'm really glad you came in. I can tell this has been stressful. *(connection)*

Patient:
It has… I've been really worried about what this could be.

Provider:
That makes complete sense. I'm here with you. *(warmth)*

Patient:
Thank you…

Patient:
So, what do you think is going on?

Provider:

It's hard to say… it could be a number of things. *(uncertain competence)*

Patient:
Like what?

Provider:
We'll just have to see how it develops. *(no clear direction)*

Patient:
That doesn't make me feel very confident…

(Internal shift begins)

Provider:
But you're not alone—I'll support you through this. *(continued connection)*

Patient:
I appreciate that…

(Patient thinking:
"They're very nice… but I'm not sure they can help me.")

Patient:
Is there anything we should be doing right now?

Provider:
Let's not rush into anything. *(softness without leadership)*

Patient:
I feel like we need a plan…

(Connection now feels hollow—not insincere, but lacking substance)

The scenario continues from the same point, but now the provider responds with a clearer, more grounded standard.

Provider:
I want to support you, and I also want to be clear about how we move forward. *(connection + competence)*

Patient:
Okay…

Provider:
Based on what I'm seeing, there are a few likely causes, and here's how we'll sort them out. *(clarity + structure)*

Patient:
That already makes me feel better.

Provider:
The next step is to run specific tests so we can get clear answers, and I'll guide you through each part. *(direction + leadership)*

Patient:
Now I feel like there's a plan.

Provider:
You deserve both support and clear guidance—and I'll make sure you have both. *(integration)*

Patient:
Now I don't just feel cared for... I feel confident in you.

When Competence Feels Inaccessible

Consider a provider who is highly knowledgeable, precise, and efficient. Their clinical decisions are sound. Their reasoning is correct. But they speak quickly. They interrupt. They explain without checking understanding. They maintain minimal eye contact.

From the provider's perspective, the encounter is successful. From the patient's perspective, something is missing. Not because the information was incorrect, but because it did not feel accessible.

Patients do not experience competence as a set of facts. They experience it as something they can understand, trust, and emotionally tolerate. If your knowledge does not reach the patient in a way they can receive, it does not fully register as competence. It registers as distance.

Dialogue: When Competence Feels Inaccessible

Provider:
Your labs indicate a mild elevation in inflammatory markers, likely consistent with a non-specific systemic response. *(technically correct, inaccessible)*

Patient:
I'm sorry... what does that mean?

Provider:
It's not uncommon. We'll monitor and reassess. *(fast, minimal engagement)*

Patient:
Is it serious?

Provider:
Not necessarily. It depends on progression. *(vague, no check for understanding)*

Patient:
I'm still confused...

Provider:
We'll repeat labs in a few weeks. *(directive, no connection)*

Patient:
Okay… I guess.

(Patient leaves uncertain, not because the care was wrong—but because it felt distant)

The scenario continues from the same point, but now the provider responds with a clearer, more grounded standard.

Provider:
Let me walk through your results in a way that's clear. *(slows down, invites understanding)*

Patient:
I'd appreciate that.

Provider:
One of your markers is slightly elevated, which can happen when your body is reacting to something like inflammation. *(translates knowledge)*

Patient:
Okay, that makes more sense.

Patient:
Is that dangerous?

Provider:
Right now, it doesn't suggest anything urgent, but it's something we should keep an eye on. *(clear, balanced)*

Patient:
That's reassuring.

Provider:
I want to pause for a moment—does this explanation feel clear so far? *(checks understanding)*

Patient:
Yes, much clearer.

Provider:
The next step is to repeat the labs in a few weeks to see if things settle down or change. *(structured plan)*

Patient:
I like knowing what comes next.

Provider:
And if anything feels off before then, I want you to reach out so we can address it early.

(accessible support)

Patient:
Thank you… now I feel like I understand what's going on.

Provider:
My goal isn't just to know the answer—it's to make sure it makes sense to you. *(competence made accessible)*

Patient:
That makes all the difference.

When Connection Feels Insufficient

Now consider the opposite. A provider who is warm, attentive, and compassionate. They listen carefully. They validate the patient's concerns. They create a sense of comfort. But their explanations are vague. Their plan lacks clarity. Their confidence appears uncertain.

The patient may feel cared for but not guided. And without guidance, care begins to feel incomplete. Connection without competence creates reassurance in the moment, but anxiety afterward.

The patient leaves thinking: *They were kind… but do they really know what they're doing?*

Dialogue: When Connection Feels Insufficient

Provider:
I'm really glad you came in. I can see how much this has been bothering you. *(strong connection)*

Patient:
It has… I've been really worried about these symptoms.

Provider:
That makes complete sense. Anyone would feel this way. *(validation)*

Patient:
Thank you…

Patient:
So, what do you think is going on?

Provider:
It's hard to say… it could be a few different things. *(vague explanation)*

Patient:
Like what kinds of things?

Provider:
Just different possibilities. We'll see how it goes. *(lacks clarity)*

Patient:

That's a little unsettling…

(Patient feels heard—but not guided)

Provider:
But you're not alone. I'll be here for you. *(continued warmth)*

Patient:
I appreciate that…

Patient (thinking):
They're kind… but I'm not sure they know what they're doing.

Patient:
Is there anything we should be doing right now?

Provider:
Let's not rush into anything. *(no direction)*

Patient:
I feel like I need a plan…

(Connection begins to feel insufficient—not because it's insincere, but because it lacks guidance)

The scenario continues from the same point, but now the provider responds with a clearer, more grounded standard.

Provider:
I want to support you, and I also want to be clear about what we're seeing and what we'll do next. *(connection + competence)*

Patient:
Okay…

Provider:
Based on your symptoms, there are a few likely causes I'm considering, and here's how we'll sort them out. *(clarity)*

Patient:
That helps a lot.

Provider:
The next step is to run specific tests so we can get clear answers, and I'll guide you through each part. *(structure + direction)*

Patient:
Now I feel like there's a plan.

Provider:

You deserve both care and clear guidance, and I'll make sure you have both. *(integration)*

Patient:
Now I don't just feel cared for... I feel confident moving forward.

The Collapse of Distinction

This is where the distinction collapses. Patients do not say: "I trust their connection, but not their competence." They say: "I'm not sure I trust them." or "I feel good about them." The mind merges both elements into a single judgment. This merging is not a flaw in patient thinking. It is a reflection of human psychology. In vulnerable situations, people rely on integrated impressions, not segmented analysis. They need to feel both safe and guided. Not one or the other.

Dialogue: The Collapse of Distinction

Provider:
I've reviewed your results. There's nothing immediately alarming. *(competence)*

Patient:
That's good to hear...

Provider:
You should follow the treatment plan I outlined. *(directive, minimal connection)*

Patient:
Okay...

Patient (thinking)**:**
They seem knowledgeable... but I don't feel comfortable.

Provider:
Do you have any questions? *(routine, detached)*

Patient:
Not really...

(Patient leaves unsure—not because competence is lacking, but because connection is missing)

In the next scenario, the situation repeats, but this time the missing element isn't connection—it's clarity.

Provider:
I understand how stressful this has been for you. *(connection)*

Patient:
It really has.

Provider:

We'll get through this together. *(warmth)*

Patient:
Thank you…

Patient:
So, what do you think is going on?

Provider:
It's hard to say… we'll see how things go. *(unclear competence)*

Patient:
That doesn't make me feel confident…

Patient (thinking):
They're nice… but I'm not sure I trust them.

In both cases, the mind merges the experience into one judgment: trust or no trust. In the final scenario, nothing about the situation changes—only the provider's ability to bring both elements together.

Provider:
I can see how much this has been weighing on you, and I want to make sure you feel both supported and clear about what's happening. *(connection + intent)*

Patient:
I appreciate that.

Provider:
Based on your results, there are a few likely causes, and here's how we're going to sort them out step by step. *(competence + structure)*

Patient:
That helps me understand.

Provider:
Right now, nothing suggests an immediate danger, but it's important we follow through carefully. *(balanced clarity)*

Patient:
That reassures me.

Provider:
My role is to both support you and guide you, so you feel confident moving forward. *(integration)*

Patient:
Now I don't just feel comfortable—I trust you.

The Emotional Interpretation of Competence

Competence is not judged only by what you know. It is judged by how you communicate what you know. Clarity signals mastery. Calmness signals control. Structure signals understanding. But so does attentiveness. When you listen without interrupting, patients interpret that as thoroughness. When you pause before answering, they interpret that as thoughtfulness. When you acknowledge uncertainty clearly, they interpret that as honesty—not weakness.

In contrast, rushed explanations feel careless. Overly technical language feels distancing. Avoiding eye contact feels uncertain. Even if the clinical reasoning is sound, the emotional signal contradicts it. And the emotional signal often wins.

Dialogue: The Emotional Interpretation of Competence

Provider:
Your results indicate a benign etiology with no immediate intervention required. *(technically correct, but distant)*

Patient:
I'm not sure I understand...

Provider:
It's nothing concerning. *(brief, rushed)*

Patient:
Okay...

Provider:
Just follow up if anything changes. *(minimal engagement)*

Patient:
...Alright.

(Patient thinking: They seemed rushed... I'm not sure how confident they really are.)

The scenario continues from the same point, but now the provider responds with a clearer, more grounded standard.

Provider:
Let me walk you through your results in a clear way. *(clarity signals mastery)*

Patient:
I'd appreciate that.

Provider:
What we're seeing is something benign, which means it isn't harmful. *(translation of knowledge)*

Patient:
Okay, that helps.

Provider:
I'm going to pause for a moment—does that make sense so far? *(checks understanding)*

Patient:
Yes, it does.

Provider:
Based on this, there's no need for immediate treatment, but we'll keep an eye on it. *(structure signals understanding)*

Patient:
That reassures me.

Patient:
So, you're confident it's not serious?

Provider:
Yes, based on what we know right now, there's nothing suggesting a serious issue. *(calm confidence)*

Patient:
That makes me feel better.

Provider:
If anything changes, I want you to reach out so we can reassess quickly. *(clear plan)*

Patient:
I like knowing that.

Provider:
I also want you to know I'm here to answer anything that feels unclear or concerning. *(attentiveness)*

Patient:
Thank you… I feel like you really took the time to explain it.

Provider:
My goal is not just to understand your condition, but to make sure you understand it too. *(competence made visible)*

Patient:
Now I feel both reassured and confident in what you're saying.

The Role of Confidence

Confidence is one of the most powerful bridges between competence and connection. But it is frequently misunderstood. Confidence is not dominance. It is not speed. It is not certainty in every answer.

True clinical confidence is quiet. It is reflected in a steady tone. A willingness to explain. An ability to say, "Here's what we know, and here's what we're going to do next."

Patients are not expecting perfection. They are looking for direction. When you provide that direction clearly and calmly, competence and connection align.

Dialogue: The Role of Confidence (Quiet, Steady, Guiding)

Patient:
I've been really anxious about these symptoms.

Provider:
It might be something, but I'm not sure yet... *(uncertainty without structure)*

Patient:
That makes me more worried.

Provider:
We'll just have to see what happens. *(passive, no direction)*

Patient:
I was hoping for a clearer answer...

(Competence may exist, but when confidence is not communicated, trust weakens)

The scenario continues from the same point, but now the provider responds with a clearer, more grounded standard.

Provider:
I can understand why this feels unsettling. Let's go through it step by step. *(steady tone + connection)*

Patient:
Okay...

Provider:
Based on what we know so far, there are a few likely explanations. *(clarity)*

Patient:
That helps.

Provider:
Here's what we know right now: nothing suggests an immediate danger. *(calm, grounded confidence)*

Patient:
That's reassuring.

Provider:
And here's what we're going to do next—we'll run specific tests to get a clear answer. *(direction)*

Patient:

Good, I needed that.

Patient:
So, you're not completely sure yet?

Provider:
We don't have the full answer yet, but we have a clear path to get there. *(confidence without over certainty)*

Patient:
That makes me feel more at ease.

Provider:
I'm going to stay with you through this process and make sure each step is clear *(guidance + presence)*

Patient:
I appreciate that.

Provider:
My goal is to give you both clarity and a steady plan forward. *(confidence defined)*

Patient:
That makes me feel like I can trust this.

Provider:
We'll take this one step at a time, and I'll make sure nothing feels uncertain or unsupported. *(connection anchored in competence)*

Patient:
Thank you... I feel much more grounded now.

Listening as a Marker of Expertise

One of the most overlooked truths in medicine is this: Patients interpret listening as a form of competence. When you allow a patient to speak without interruption, they do not just feel respected. They feel that you are gathering information thoroughly. When you reflect back what they have said, they do not just feel heard. They feel that you understand their case. Listening is not separate from diagnosis. It is part of it, and patients sense that.

Dialogue: Listening as a Marker of Expertise

Patient:
I've been having these headaches, and they seem to be getting worse.

Provider:
How long have you had them? *(quick, task-focused)*

Patient:
About a month, but—

Provider:
Any nausea or vision changes? *(interrupts, checklist mode)*

Patient:
Sometimes, but I was also—

Provider:
We'll likely need imaging to rule things out. *(premature conclusion)*

Patient:
I don't feel like I explained everything…

(Patient thinking:
They didn't really listen… are they missing something?)

The scenario continues from the same point, but now the provider responds with a clearer, more grounded standard.

Provider:
Tell me more about the headaches—start wherever it makes the most sense to you. *(invites full narrative)*

Patient:
They started about a month ago, but lately they've been more frequent, especially in the mornings.

Provider:
I'm hearing that they've been increasing and are worse in the morning. *(reflects back)*

Patient:
Yes, exactly.

Patient:
I've also been feeling more tired than usual.

Provider:
That's important—headaches and fatigue together give us more to think about. *(integrates information)*

Patient:
I'm glad you're taking that into account.

Provider:
I want to make sure I have the full picture—anything else you've noticed, even if it seems unrelated? *(encourages completeness)*

Patient:
Sometimes my vision feels a little blurry.

Provider:
That's very helpful to know. *(affirms contribution)*

Patient:
I wasn't sure if it mattered.

Provider:
It does. The more complete the picture, the better we can understand what's going on. *(links listening to competence)*

Patient:
That makes sense.

Provider:
Based on everything you've shared, I have a clearer sense of what we should evaluate next. *(demonstrates thoroughness)*

Patient:
I feel like you really understand what I'm dealing with.

Provider:
Listening carefully helps me make better decisions—and helps us get to the right answer together. *(listening framed as expertise)*

Patient:
That makes me feel confident in you.

The Danger of Imbalance

When providers lean too heavily on one side, the imbalance becomes visible. Competence without connection feels cold, distant, and sometimes arrogant. Connection without competence feels warm, but uncertain and incomplete. Neither builds durable trust. The goal is not to choose between them. It is to integrate them so seamlessly that the patient cannot distinguish where one ends and the other begins.

Dialogue: The Danger of Imbalance

Provider:
Your test results confirm a mild cardiac arrhythmia. We'll start medication and monitor response. *(competence without connection)*

Patient:
That sounds serious…

Provider:
It's manageable. Just follow the plan. *(efficient, but cold)*

Patient:
I still feel worried…

Provider:
There's no need to worry. *(dismissive reassurance)*

Patient:
...Okay.

(Patient thinking:
They know what they're doing... but I don't feel comfortable.)

In the next scenario, the situation repeats, but this time the missing element isn't connection—it's clarity.

Provider:
I can see how scary this must feel for you. *(connection without competence)*

Patient:
It really is...

Provider:
You're not alone. I'm here with you. *(warmth)*

Patient:
Thank you...

Patient:
So, what does this mean?

Provider:
It's hard to say exactly... we'll see how things go. *(lacks clarity)*

Patient:
That doesn't make me feel confident...

(Patient thinking:
They're kind... but I'm not sure they know what they're doing.)

In both cases, trust remains incomplete. In the final scenario, nothing about the situation changes—only the provider's ability to bring both elements together.

Provider:
I can see how concerning this is, and I want to walk you through it clearly. *(connection + clarity)*

Patient:
Okay...

Provider:
Your results show an irregular heart rhythm. The good news is that it's something we can manage effectively. *(competence explained clearly)*

Patient:
That helps me understand.

Provider:
The next step is to start medication and monitor how your body responds. *(direction)*

Patient:
I like knowing what comes next.

Provider:
I'll guide you through this so nothing feels uncertain, and we'll adjust as needed. *(leadership + support)*

Patient:
That makes me feel both supported and confident.

Provider:
My goal is for you to feel not only cared for but also clear about every step we take. *(integration)*

Patient:
Now I trust both what you're saying and how you're guiding me.

The Internal Alignment

For providers of healthcare delivery, this integration begins internally. If you view connection as an "extra," it will feel optional in practice. If you view competence as purely technical, it will feel disconnected from the patient experience. But when you understand that connection is the vehicle through which competence is delivered, your approach changes. You begin to see:

- Explaining clearly is part of being competent.
- Listening fully is part of being competent.
- Creating emotional safety is part of being competent.

Not additions. Essentials.

Dialogue: The Internal Alignment

Provider:
Your condition is stable. Continue your current regimen. *(competence as purely technical)*

Patient:
Okay... what does "stable" really mean for me?

Provider:
It means it's not getting worse. *(minimal explanation)*

Patient:
I'm still not sure I understand...

(Patient leaves with information, but without clarity or confidence. Provider reflects and shifts internal approach.)

Provider:
Let me explain what "stable" means in a way that's clear for you. *(explaining as competence)*

Patient:
I'd appreciate that.

Provider:
It means your condition hasn't worsened, which is a positive sign, and we want to keep it that way. *(clarity)*

Patient:
That makes more sense.

Provider:
I also want to hear how you've been feeling day to day. *(listening as competence)*

Patient:
I've been better, but still worried sometimes.

Provider:
That's important to know. Your experience helps guide how we manage this. *(integration of listening)*

Patient:
I'm glad you asked.

Provider:
The next step is to continue your current treatment and monitor closely so we can adjust if needed. *(structured plan)*

Patient:
I like knowing there's a plan.

Provider:
I want you to feel comfortable asking anything that's unclear—that's part of how we make good decisions together. *(emotional safety as competence)*

Patient:
That makes me feel more at ease.

Provider:
My goal is not just to know your condition, but to make sure you understand it and feel supported managing it. *(internal alignment expressed)*

Patient:
Now I feel like you really know what you're doing—and that you care.

What Patients Actually Remember

Patients rarely leave an encounter thinking in technical terms. They do not recall differential diagnoses or clinical reasoning pathways. They remember something much simpler: *"Did I feel confident in this doctor?"* And that confidence is built from both what you did and how you made them feel.

Dialogue: What Patients Actually Remember (Refined)

Provider:
Based on your symptoms, we're considering a differential that includes a viral process versus an early inflammatory condition.

Patient:
I'm not sure I understand…

Provider:
We'll run some labs and reassess once we have more information.

Patient:
Okay…

Provider:
Any questions?

Patient:
Not really…

(Patient leaves with appropriate care—but without confidence. Later thought: "I don't know… something didn't feel clear.")

In the next scenario, nothing about the medical decision changes — only the clarity and structure the provider brings to the moment.

Provider:
I want to walk you through what I'm thinking in a way that makes sense.

Patient:
Thank you.

Provider:
Based on your symptoms, there are a couple of likely causes. The good news is that most of them are manageable.

Patient:
That's reassuring.

Provider:
The next step is to run some straightforward tests so we can be certain and choose the right treatment.

Patient:
That makes sense.

Provider:
I also want to make sure I'm addressing what's worrying you most—what's been on your mind?

Patient:
I was afraid it might be something serious.

Provider:
I understand that concern. Right now, nothing suggests anything immediately dangerous, but we'll evaluate it carefully so we're sure.

Patient:
That really helps.

Provider:
I'll guide you through each step, so you always know what we're doing and why.

Patient:
I appreciate that.

(Patient leaves with the same clinical plan—but a different internal experience. Later thought: "I felt confident in them.")

A Higher Standard

To practice at the highest level requires more than mastering medical knowledge. It requires mastering how that knowledge is experienced by another human being. This is the point where medicine becomes more than science; it becomes relational. And in that relationship, competence and connection are not competing forces; they are partners. Each incomplete without the other. Each strengthening the other when aligned.

Dialogue: A Higher Standard

Provider:
Your imaging confirms a benign lesion. No intervention is required at this time. *(technically correct)*

Patient:
Okay… is that something I should be worried about?

Provider:
No, it's benign. We'll just monitor it. *(efficient, but limited connection)*

Patient:
Alright…

(Patient leaves with accurate information, but lingering uncertainty. Later thought: "I guess it's okay… but I'm not completely sure.")

In the next scenario, nothing about the findings changes — only the standard the provider brings to the explanation.

Provider:
I want to go over your results in a way that feels clear and reassuring. *(relational intent)*

Patient:
Thank you.

Provider:
The imaging shows something called a benign lesion, which means it's not harmful. *(competence translated)*

Patient:
That's a relief.

Provider:
Right now, there's no need for treatment, but we'll monitor it over time to make sure it stays that way. *(structure + direction)*

Patient:
That makes sense.

Provider:
I also want to check in—what concerns did you have coming into this visit? *(connection)*

Patient:
I was worried it might be cancer.

Provider:
I understand that fear. Based on what we see, there's nothing suggesting that. *(clarity + reassurance)*

Patient:
That really helps.

Provider:
My goal is not just to interpret the results, but to make sure you feel confident in what they mean for you. *(higher standard expressed)*

Patient:
I can feel that.

Provider:
Medicine isn't just about having the right answer—it's about making sure that answer reaches you in a way that feels clear and steady. *(integration)*

Patient:
That makes me trust what you're saying even more.

Provider:
When both are aligned, you don't just leave with information—you leave with confidence.
(conclusion embodied)

Patient:
That's exactly how I feel right now.

Closing Reflection

Before your next patient encounter, consider not just what you need to know—but how it will be received. Ask yourself:

Will this patient understand me?

Will they feel guided?

Will they feel that I am both capable and present?

Because in the patient's mind, there is no separation. There is only one conclusion: *"This is someone I trust."*

Chapter 3

The Hidden Curriculum in Medicine

What Students Absorb But Are Never Formally Taught

There are two educational programs taking place in medical school. One is explicit. It is structured, examined, and carefully outlined. It lives in lectures, textbooks, clinical guidelines, and standardized assessments. It teaches anatomy, physiology, pathology, and pharmacology. It defines what students are expected to know.

The other is unspoken. It is not written in the syllabus. It is not tested on exams. It is not formally acknowledged. And yet, it is often more powerful. This is the hidden curriculum. It is the set of behaviors, attitudes, priorities, and emotional habits that students absorb simply by being present in the medical environment. It is learned through observation, imitation, and repeated exposure. And it answers a different question than the formal curriculum: not "What should I know?" but "How am I supposed to be."

Learning Without Being Taught

From the first day of clinical exposure, students begin watching. They watch how healthcare providers enter rooms. They watch how they speak to patients—and how they speak about patients. They watch what is prioritized and what is ignored. They watch how time is managed, how stress is handled, how uncertainty is expressed or concealed.

No one formally instructs them to internalize these patterns. But they do. Because in complex, high-pressure environments, human beings learn by modeling. When uncertainty is high, we look to those with authority and experience to define what is "normal," what is "acceptable," and what is "expected." And in medicine, those definitions are rarely spoken directly. They are demonstrated.

The Messages Beneath the Surface

The hidden curriculum is not a single lesson. It is a collection of repeated signals that, over time, form a coherent belief system. Students begin to absorb messages such as:

- Efficiency is valued more than presence
- Emotional distance is a form of professionalism

- Vulnerability should be concealed
- Difficult conversations should be shortened when possible
- Technical accuracy matters more than relational depth
- Time spent connecting is time taken away from productivity

These messages are rarely stated explicitly. In fact, they often contradict what is taught in formal lectures about empathy, communication, and patient-centered care. This creates a quiet but powerful conflict. Students are told one thing. They observe another. And over time, what they observe tends to win.

The Power of Repetition

A single observation does not shape behavior; repetition does. When a student repeatedly sees healthcare providers interrupt patients, they begin to view interruption as efficient rather than dismissive. When they see minimal eye contact paired with effective diagnoses, they begin to believe that connection is optional. When they observe senior healthcare providers moving quickly from room to room without pause, they begin to equate speed with competence. These patterns accumulate. They do not feel like choices. They begin to feel like standards.

Emotional Adaptation

The hidden curriculum does not only shape behavior. It shapes emotional responses. Students enter medicine with a wide range of emotional capacities. Many are empathetic, attentive, and deeply motivated to connect with patients. But they quickly encounter an environment where emotional exposure is constant and often intense: suffering, uncertainty, loss, pressure.

Without structured guidance on how to process these experiences, students adapt. And the most common adaptation is emotional distancing. Not because they do not care, but because they are not shown how to care sustainably. Over time, this distancing can become normalized. It begins to feel like maturity, professionalism, or resilience. But in many cases, it is simply unaddressed emotional fatigue.

Language as a Teaching Tool

One of the most powerful components of the hidden curriculum is language. How healthcare providers speak about patients, especially outside the room, leaves a lasting impression. A patient becomes "the gallbladder in room 4," a complex individual becomes "a difficult case," and a person in distress becomes "non-compliant."

This language is efficient. It is shorthand. It serves a functional purpose in fast-paced environments, but it also subtly reshapes perception. It reduces complexity, creates distance and shifts focus from the person to the problem. Students absorb this language and, with it, the mindset that accompanies it. Without realizing it, they begin to see patients less as individuals and more as clinical scenarios.

The Disappearance of Reflection

In the formal curriculum, reflection is encouraged. Students are asked to think about their experiences, to process difficult encounters and to consider the emotional dimensions of care. In the clinical environment, reflection often disappears. There is little time, little structure and little modeling.

Encounters happen in rapid succession. There is no pause to ask:

- What just happened in that room?
- How did the patient experience that interaction?
- What could have been done differently?

Without reflection, experiences are not processed. They are simply accumulated. And what is accumulated without examination becomes habit.

The Unintended Consequence

The hidden curriculum does not exist because healthcare providers intend to teach it. It exists because systems prioritize efficiency, volume, and measurable outcomes, often at the expense of relational depth. Healthcare providers themselves are operating under pressure: time constraints, administrative demands, cognitive load. In that environment, behaviors become streamlined. Conversations shorten, nonverbal connection decreases and emotional engagement becomes selective.

Students are not witnessing idealized medicine. They are witnessing practiced medicine under constraint, and they learn accordingly.

The Risk to Future Practice

If left unexamined, the hidden curriculum shapes not only how students behave, but how they define good care. They may begin to believe that:

- Connection is optional
- Efficiency is the primary marker of skill
- Emotional neutrality is preferable to engagement
- Communication is secondary to decision-making

These beliefs do not develop suddenly; they form gradually through exposure. Once formed, they are difficult to reverse.

Awareness as the First Intervention

The hidden curriculum cannot be eliminated entirely. But it can be made visible. Awareness changes how students interpret what they observe. Instead of absorbing behaviors automatically, they begin to evaluate them:

- Is this efficient, or is it dismissive?
- Is this professionalism, or is it emotional avoidance?
- Is this clarity, or is it oversimplification?

This shift from passive absorption to active interpretation is critical. It allows students to choose what they carry forward.

Reclaiming Intentional Practice

To counterbalance the hidden curriculum, students must become intentional about their development. This means actively practicing:

- Maintaining eye contact, even when others do not
- Listening fully, even when time feels limited
- Explaining clearly, even when brevity is encouraged
- Acknowledging emotion, even when it is uncomfortable

These are not acts of resistance; they are acts of alignment. They align the healthcare provider you are becoming with the healthcare provider you intended to be.

The Role of Mentorship

Not all elements of the hidden curriculum are negative. There are healthcare providers who model presence, clarity, and respect consistently, even within constrained systems. When students encounter these individuals, something important happens: they see that it is possible—possible to be efficient and present, to be competent and connected, to maintain humanity without sacrificing performance. These healthcare providers may not formally teach these qualities, but they demonstrate them, and demonstration, in medicine, is one of the most powerful forms of teaching.

Closing Reflection

At some point in your training, you will realize that you are no longer just learning medicine. You are becoming a healthcare provider. That process is shaped not only by what you are taught, but by what you absorb. The hidden curriculum will influence you whether you acknowledge it or not. The question is not whether it exists. The question is whether you will remain aware of it. Because the kind of healthcare provider you become will not be determined solely by your knowledge. It will be determined by the standards you adopt—consciously or unconsciously—along the way. And those standards begin forming long before you realize they are shaping you.

Chapter 4

Presence Over Perfection

What Patients Actually Need in Difficult Moments

There is a quiet misunderstanding at the heart of modern medicine. Many providers, from the earliest days of training through decades of practice, come to believe that their value lies primarily in precision, knowledge, and technical execution. They strive to be correct, efficient, and decisive. These are essential qualities. Lives depend on them. Yet, in the moments that matter most to patients, these are not the qualities patients remember first. Patients remember how you were with them.

Presence is often mistaken for something vague or secondary, but it is, in truth, one of the most powerful clinical tools a provider possesses. It does not require perfection. It does not demand that you have every answer. It asks only that you are fully there, attentive, engaged, and human in your interaction.

When a patient receives difficult news, they are not processing information the way a provider delivers it. Their mind fragments. Fear narrows their ability to absorb detail. In these moments, clarity of data becomes less important than clarity of connection. A perfectly delivered explanation, devoid of presence, can feel cold and alienating. An imperfect explanation, delivered with genuine attention and steadiness, can feel grounding and safe. This is the paradox: patients do not need you to be flawless. They need you to be present.

For healthcare students, this can feel counterintuitive. Training emphasizes mastery, accuracy, and avoiding error. Communication is often taught as a structured skill set, a checklist of behaviors to demonstrate competence. While these frameworks are useful, they can unintentionally create distance. Students may become so focused on "doing it right" that they stop simply being with the patient.

Presence is not a script. It is not a technique to perform. It is the willingness to slow down internally, even when time is limited, and to recognize that the person in front of you is not just a case, but someone navigating uncertainty, vulnerability, and often fear.

For experienced providers, the challenge is different. Over time, repetition can dull sensitivity. Difficult conversations become familiar. Efficiency becomes necessary. There is a natural tendency to protect oneself from emotional fatigue by creating distance. This is understandable, but it carries a cost. Patients can sense when a provider is physically present but emotionally elsewhere.

Presence does not mean absorbing every patient's pain or becoming emotionally overwhelmed. It means allowing yourself to acknowledge the weight of the moment without retreating from it. It is the ability to sit in discomfort without rushing to escape it through excessive information, premature reassurance, or clinical detachment.

Consider the difference between these two approaches. In one, a provider delivers a diagnosis quickly, explains the treatment plan thoroughly, and moves on, believing they have done their job well. In the other, the provider pauses, observes the patient's reaction, allows silence, and responds not only to the medical condition but to the emotional reality unfolding in front of them.

The second approach does not take significantly more time. It requires a shift in awareness. Patients are remarkably perceptive. They may not understand the complexities of their condition, but they understand tone, eye contact, and attention. They can tell when a provider is rushed, distracted, or disengaged. More importantly, they can tell when a provider is truly with them.

This has profound implications for trust. Trust is not built solely on competence, though competence is essential. It is built on the patient's sense that their providers see them, hear them, and care about their experience, not just their diagnosis. When presence is absent, even excellent care can feel insufficient. When presence is strong, even difficult news can be received with a sense of support and partnership.

This is what this section is about. It is not about replacing clinical excellence with emotional connection, but about recognizing that the two are inseparable in the patient's experience. It is about teaching healthcare students that communication is not an accessory to medicine, but a core component of it. It is about reminding experienced providers that, despite years of practice, the human element of care remains as important as ever.

Presence over perfection is not a lowering of standards. It is a refinement of priorities. You will not always have the right words. You will not always be able to fix what is wrong but you can always choose how you show up in the moment. For the patient, that choice often matters more than anything you say.

What follows is a brief example that illustrates the difference.

Dialogue 1: Focused on Perfection (Technically Correct, Emotionally Distant)

Provider:
Mr. Lewis, your biopsy confirms adenocarcinoma of the pancreas.

Patient:
...Cancer?

Provider:
Yes. Based on staging, it appears to be at least Stage II, possibly III pending imaging.

Patient:
I... I don't understand what that means.

Provider:
It means the tumor has likely extended beyond the pancreas. We'll need a CT scan to confirm vascular involvement.

Patient:
Is it… treatable?

Provider:
Treatment typically involves chemotherapy, possibly followed by surgical evaluation depending on respectability.

Patient:
Am I going to die?

Provider:
Prognosis varies. Median survival rates depend on staging and response to treatment.

Patient:
This is a lot…

Provider:
I understand. I'll have oncology schedule you. They'll go over the protocol in detail.

Patient:
…Okay.

Provider:
Do you have any other questions about the treatment plan?

Dialogue 2: Focused on Presence (Human Connection with Clinical Clarity)

Provider:
Mr. Lewis… I have your biopsy results. It does show cancer in the pancreas.

Patient:
…Cancer?

Provider:
Yes. I'm really sorry. I can see this is a lot to take in.

Patient:
I don't even know what to think right now.

Provider:
That makes sense. Most people feel overwhelmed hearing this. We can go through it slowly, together.

Patient:
Is it… bad?

Provider:
It is serious, but there are treatments, and we'll walk through each step carefully. You won't be facing this alone.

Patient:
Am I going to die?

Provider:
I hear how scary that question is. What I can tell you is that we'll focus on giving you the best care possible and supporting you through this.

Patient:
I'm just... scared.

Provider:
Of course you are. Anyone would be. We can take a moment if you need. I'm here with you.

Patient:
...Thank you.

Provider:
When you're ready, I can explain what this means and what the next steps look like, one piece at a time.

Part II

Communication That Builds or Breaks Trust

Chapter 5	The First Conversation	64
Chapter 6	Listening Beyond Symptoms	70
Chapter 7	Words That Land—and Words That Harm	75
Chapter 8	The 10-Minute Rule — Creating Meaningful Connections Even in Limited Time	98

Chapter 5

The First Conversation

Setting Tone, Safety, and Credibility

The first conversation between a provider and a patient is not simply an introduction. It is a defining moment. Within minutes, often within seconds, patients begin forming conclusions that will shape how they interpret everything that follows. Before they fully understand your credentials, your treatment plan, or even their diagnosis, they are asking themselves quieter, more instinctive questions: *Am I safe here? Does this person see me? Can I trust them?*

These questions are not answered through medical knowledge. They are answered through presence, tone, and subtle human signals that are often overlooked in clinical training.

Tone is established before words are fully processed. The way you enter the room, the pace of your movements, whether you sit or stand, whether your attention feels divided or focused—these elements communicate far more than the content of your speech. A rushed entrance, even with the best intentions, signals urgency and distance. A brief pause, eye contact, and a grounded posture signal availability. Patients may not consciously register these details, but they feel them immediately.

Tone also lives in your voice. A provider who speaks quickly, clinically, and without modulation may sound efficient but can feel inaccessible. In contrast, a measured, steady tone conveys control without detachment. It tells the patient: *There is time for you here, even if the schedule is full.*

Safety is emotional before it is clinical. In medicine, safety is often defined in terms of avoiding errors, following protocols, and ensuring correct treatment. But from the patient's perspective, safety begins at a different level. It begins with whether they feel comfortable expressing confusion, fear, or even disagreement.

If a patient senses judgment, impatience, or dismissal, they will withhold. They may nod in agreement while internally uncertain. They may leave without asking the question that matters most. This is how miscommunication begins, not from a lack of intelligence, but from a lack of emotional safety.

Creating safety does not require long conversations. It requires small, intentional signals: a pause after delivering information, an acknowledgment of uncertainty or fear, an invitation such as, "*What concerns you most right now?*" These moments give the patient permission to participate honestly.

Credibility is not built on knowledge alone. Providers often assume that credibility is established through expertise, credentials, and clarity of explanation. While these are essential, they are not sufficient. Patients rarely have the ability to evaluate technical competence directly. Instead, they use relational cues as a proxy.

A provider who appears attentive, listens without interruption, and responds to what the patient is actually saying, not just what is medically relevant, feels more credible. Not because they necessarily are more skilled, but because they are perceived as more trustworthy.

This creates a powerful and sometimes uncomfortable truth: a highly competent provider who appears disengaged may be trusted less than a moderately competent provider who is fully present. Ideally, both qualities coexist. But when they do not, patients choose connection as their anchor.

The first conversation shapes all future conversations. If the initial interaction feels rushed or impersonal, patients carry that impression forward. They may become more guarded, less communicative, and less likely to share critical details. Trust, once weakened early, requires significant effort to rebuild.

Conversely, when the first conversation establishes warmth, attentiveness, and clarity, it creates momentum. Patients become more open, more engaged, and more likely to adhere to recommendations. The provider's job becomes easier, not harder, because the relationship itself supports the care.

This is where presence and structure must meet. The goal is not to abandon efficiency or clinical rigor. It is to integrate them with awareness. A well-structured conversation can still feel deeply human when it includes moments of pause, acknowledgment, and responsiveness.

Consider a simple framework, not as a script, but as a mindset:

1. Begin by orienting yourself to the patient, not just the chart.
2. Acknowledge the context, why they are there, and what they may be feeling.
3. Deliver information clearly, but not hurriedly.
4. Pause, observe, and respond to their reaction.
5. Invite questions in a way that feels genuine, not procedural.

Each of these steps may take only seconds, but together they transform the interaction.

For healthcare students, this is a skill that must be practiced early. It is easy to focus on memorization, diagnosis, and technical ability, believing that communication will develop naturally over time. In reality, habits form quickly. If presence is not intentionally cultivated, distance becomes the default.

For experienced providers, this is a skill that must be revisited. Years of practice can create efficiency, but it can also make you drift into autopilot. The first conversation can begin to feel routine. Yet for the patient, it is never routine. It is often one of the most important conversations of their life.

The challenge is not learning something entirely new but remembering what is easy to forget: every first conversation is, in a very real sense, a threshold moment. You are not just exchanging information; you are defining the relationship. And once that definition is set, everything that follows is shaped by it.

Demonstration: The First Conversation (Setting Tone, Safety, and Credibility)

Provider:

Good morning, Mr. Harris. I'm Dr. Patel. I'm glad you came in today.

Patient:
Morning… I wasn't sure if I should come, honestly.

Provider:
I'm really glad you did. What's been weighing on you enough to bring you in?

Patient:
I've been having this pain… and I keep thinking it might be something serious.

Provider:
That sounds unsettling. Tell me more about what the pain has been like.

Patient:
It comes and goes, but lately it's been more frequent.

Provider:
I hear that it's changing, and that's understandably concerning. When did you first notice it?

Patient:
Maybe a couple months ago… but I ignored it at first.

Provider:
A lot of people do that. You're not alone in waiting to see if it passes.

Patient:
Yeah… I guess I was hoping it would just go away.

Provider:
Of course. Anyone would hope for that. What worries you most about it right now?

Patient:
That it's something bad… like cancer or something.

Provider:
I can understand why your mind would go there. Let's take this step by step together.

Patient:
Okay…

Provider:
I'm going to ask a few more questions and then we'll decide what tests, if any, we need. Does that sound alright?

Patient:
Yes, that helps.

Provider:
And as we go, if something doesn't make sense or you have a concern, please stop me anytime.

Patient:
I appreciate that.

Provider:
You're not alone in this. We'll figure it out together.

Patient:
Thank you… that makes me feel a lot better already.

Dialogue: Language as a Clinical Tool (Second Example)

This exchange shows how a single clinical conversation can unfold along two parallel tracks: the automatic response a provider might give under pressure, and a reframed version that lands with clarity, compassion, and support.

Provider:
Your blood sugar is uncontrolled. *(harsh, judgmental tone)*

Patient:
I've been trying…

Provider:
You need to do better with your diet. *(blame-focused)*

Patient:
That's discouraging to hear.

A reframed approach shifts from blame to clarity.

Provider:
Your blood sugar levels are higher than we'd like right now. *(neutral, informative)*

Patient:
I was afraid of that…

Provider:
Managing this can be challenging. Let's look at what's been working and where we can adjust. *(supportive, collaborative)*

Patient:
I appreciate that approach.

The patient expresses shame; the automatic response reinforces it.

Patient:
I feel like I've failed at this.

Provider:
You just need more discipline. *(reinforces shame)*

Patient:
That makes me feel worse.

The reframed response removes blame and restores perspective.

Provider:
This isn't about failure. Many people struggle with this, and we can work through it together. *(removes blame)*

Patient:
That helps me feel less alone.

The automatic response uses fear; the patient absorbs the threat.

Provider:
If you don't control this, you'll have complications. *(fear-based, threatening)*

Patient:
That scares me…

The reframed version offers information without fear.

Provider:
Keeping your blood sugar in range helps reduce the risk of complications, and we can take steps to move in that direction. *(informative without fear)*

Patient:
That feels more manageable.

The patient asks for guidance; the automatic response oversimplifies.

Patient:
What should I do next?

Provider:
Cut out sugar and exercise more. *(oversimplified, directive)*

Patient:
I've tried that before…

The reframed response focuses on realistic, individualized change.

Provider:
Let's find one or two changes that fit realistically into your routine, so it doesn't feel overwhelming.

(practical, individualized)

Patient:
I think I can do that.

The automatic close feels transactional.

Provider:
Come back in three months. *(transactional close)*

Patient:
Okay ...

The reframed close reinforces ongoing support.

Provider:
We'll follow up in three months, but if anything feels difficult before then, I want you to reach out so we can adjust together. *(ongoing support)*

Patient:
Thank you... that makes me feel supported.

Chapter 6

Listening Beyond Symptoms

Hearing fear, Not Just Facts.

In medicine, listening is often assumed to be a basic skill, something that naturally occurs as part of taking a history. Questions are asked, answers are recorded, and patterns are identified. From a clinical standpoint, this process is efficient and necessary. But from the patient's perspective, this version of listening can feel incomplete.

Patients rarely come in with symptoms alone. They come with interpretations, fears, assumptions, and personal narratives that shape how those symptoms are experienced. If a provider listens only for data, they may capture what is happening but miss the meaning. And it is often the meaning that determines how a patient responds to care.

Listening beyond symptoms requires a shift in attention. Instead of focusing solely on extracting information, the provider begins to notice how the patient tells their story. What do they emphasize? What do they repeat? Where do they hesitate? These subtle cues often reveal more than the words themselves.

A patient describing chest pain may be speaking about more than physical discomfort. Beneath the description may be fear of a heart attack, anxiety about family responsibilities, or even guilt over lifestyle choices. If the provider responds only to the symptom, ordering tests and explaining probabilities, the deeper concern remains unaddressed. The patient may leave with answers, but without reassurance.

This is where many interactions fall short. The provider believes they have listened because they have gathered accurate information. The patient feels unheard because what mattered most to them was never acknowledged.

True listening involves recognizing both layers simultaneously. It means hearing the clinical content while also attending to the emotional undercurrent. This does not require long conversations or dramatic expressions of empathy. Often, it is as simple as naming what is already present: "You've mentioned this pain several times—it sounds like it's really been on your mind." or "You seem worried this could be something serious." These statements do not slow the visit significantly, but they change its quality. They signal to the patient that their internal experience has been seen, not just their external symptoms.

Another important dimension of listening is restraint. Providers are trained to think quickly, to form differential diagnoses, and to guide conversations efficiently. While this is essential, it can lead to premature interruption. Studies have shown that patients are often interrupted within seconds of beginning to speak. When this happens, important information is lost, not just medically but relationally.

Allowing a patient to complete their initial thought, even if it takes an extra minute, often leads to greater clarity and fewer misunderstandings later. More importantly, it builds trust. The patient senses that their voice matters.

Listening beyond symptoms also means tolerating moments of ambiguity. Not every pause needs to be filled. Not every silence is a problem to solve. Sometimes, a patient is gathering the courage to say something difficult. If the provider rushes to the next question, that moment is lost.

For healthcare students, this can feel uncomfortable. Silence can feel like inaction. There is a temptation to fill it with more questions, more structure, more control. But with experience, it becomes clear that some of the most important information emerges in these unstructured moments.

For experienced providers, the challenge is different. Familiarity can create assumptions. After hearing similar complaints hundreds of times, it is easy to anticipate the story before it is fully told. This can lead to subtle forms of disengagement, finishing sentences, redirecting prematurely, or overlooking unique aspects of the patient's experience.

Each patient, however, is encountering their situation for the first time. What feels routine to the provider is often significant to them.

Listening beyond symptoms is not about abandoning efficiency or clinical reasoning. It is about expanding awareness. It is the ability to gather accurate medical information while also understanding the person who is living with it.

When patients feel truly heard, several things happen. They become more open. They share more accurate information. They are more likely to follow recommendations. And perhaps most importantly, they feel less alone in what they are experiencing.

In the end, listening is not just a diagnostic tool. It is a form of care in itself. And when done well, it transforms not only what the provider understands, but what the patient experiences internally as they navigate their care.

Conversation 1: Listening Only to Symptoms (Data Collected, Meaning Missed)

Provider:
What brings you in today?

Patient:
I've been having chest pain on and off.

Provider:
Where exactly is the pain located?

Patient:
Right here, kind of in the center.

Provider:
Does it radiate anywhere?

Patient:
Sometimes to my left arm.

Provider:
How long does it last?

Patient:
Maybe a few minutes each time.

Provider:
Any shortness of breath?

Patient:
A little, yes.

Provider:
Any nausea or sweating?

Patient:
Sometimes sweating.

Provider:
Do you have a history of heart disease?

Patient:
No, but—

Provider:
Do you smoke?

Patient:
I used to.

Provider:
We'll need an EKG and some blood work to rule out cardiac causes.

Patient:
Okay…

Provider:
Avoid exertion until we have results.

Patient:
I've been really worried it might be something serious…

Provider:
We'll evaluate that after the tests.

Patient:
...Alright.

Conversation 2: Listening Beyond Symptoms (Data + Meaning Understood)

Provider:
What brings you in today?

Patient:
I've been having chest pain on and off.

Provider:
That sounds concerning. Tell me what it's been like for you.

Patient:
It's right in the center, and sometimes it goes to my arm.

Provider:
I'm hearing both the location and that it spreads—when did this start?

Patient:
A few weeks ago... but it's happening more now.

Provider:
That change alone can feel unsettling. What's been going through your mind when it happens?

Patient:
Honestly... I keep thinking it might be a heart attack.

Provider:
That's a heavy thought to carry. It makes sense that you'd be worried.

Patient:
Yeah, I haven't really told anyone how scared I've been.

Provider:
I'm really glad you shared that with me. We'll take this seriously and look at it carefully together.

Patient:
Okay...

Provider:
I do want to ask a few specific questions to understand the symptoms better—would that be alright?

Patient:
Yes, of course.

Provider:
When the pain comes, how long does it usually last?

Patient:
A few minutes.

Provider:
Any shortness of breath or sweating with it?

Patient:
Yes, both sometimes.

Provider:
Thank you—that helps medically, and I also hear how stressful this has been for you.

Patient:
It really has.

Provider:
We'll run tests like an EKG and labs, but just as important, I want you to know we're going to walk through this step by step so you're not carrying that fear alone.

Chapter 7

Words That Land—and Words That Harm

Subtle Language Differences with Lasting Impact

Language in medicine is often treated as a neutral vehicle, a means of transmitting information from provider to patient with clarity and efficiency. Yet in practice, words are never neutral. They carry tone, implication, hierarchy, and emotional weight. A single phrase can either steady a patient or unsettle them, build trust or quietly erode it. What is said matters, but how it is said often matters more.

For both healthcare students and experienced providers, this distinction is easy to underestimate. Clinical training prioritizes accuracy, brevity, and decisiveness. These are essential in diagnosis and treatment. But when those same habits are applied to human interaction without awareness, they can create unintended harm. Not through negligence or lack of care, but through language that misses the patient's emotional reality.

At the center of this topic is a simple but profound truth: patients do not experience words the way providers intend them. They experience words through the filter of fear, uncertainty, past experiences, and vulnerability. What feels routine to a provider may feel deeply personal to a patient.

Consider the difference between these two statements:

1. "This is a common condition."
2. "We see this often, and we have clear ways to help manage it."

Both statements convey similar information. Yet the first can feel dismissive, as if the patient's experience is being minimized. The second maintains reassurance while preserving the patient's sense of significance. The distinction is subtle, but its impact is not. This is the nature of language in medicine. Small differences carry large consequences.

Dialogue: Words That Harm vs. Words That Land

Provider:
Your test results are negative.

Patient:
Negative… is that bad?

Provider:
No, it means nothing was found. *(unclear, anxiety-provoking word choice)*

This wording is technically correct but unclear, which can heighten anxiety. A clearer alternative would be:

Provider:
The results did not show any signs of disease, which is reassuring. *(clear and reassuring)*

Patient:
I've been really worried about this.

Provider:
There's nothing to worry about. *(dismisses emotion)*

This dismisses the patient's fear. A more supportive response acknowledges the emotion first:

Provider:
I can see why this has been worrying you. Let's walk through what we know together. *(acknowledges feeling)*

Patient:
So, what happens next?

Provider:
You'll need to comply with the treatment plan. *(authoritative, distancing)*

This can feel authoritative and distancing. A collaborative alternative is:

Provider:
Let's go over the plan together so it feels manageable for you. *(collaborative tone)*

Patient:
I'm not sure I can handle all of this.

Provider:
You have to stay positive. *(minimizes struggle)*

This minimizes the patient's struggle. A more grounded response is:

Provider:
This can feel overwhelming. We can take it one step at a time. *(realistic support)*

Patient:
Did the treatment fail?

Provider:
Yes, the treatment failed. *(harsh, personal sounding)*

Stated this way, the "failure" can feel personal and harsh. A gentler, more accurate framing is:

Provider:
This treatment didn't work the way we hoped, so we'll look at other options. *(removes blame, preserves hope)*

Patient:
Is this common?

Provider:
This is a very common condition. *(can feel dismissive)*

While factual, this can sound dismissive of the patient's experience. A more reassuring alternative is:

Provider:
We see this often, and there are well-established ways to treat it. *(normalizes while reassuring)*

Patient:
I feel like I caused this.

Provider:
You should have come in sooner. *(implies blame)*

This reinforces blame and shame. A response that removes judgment and restores perspective is:

Provider:
Many people wait to see if symptoms improve. What matters is that you're here now. *(removes judgment)*

Patient:
I just don't understand everything.

Provider:
Do you understand what I said? *(can feel testing or pressured)*

This can feel like a test rather than an invitation. A more open, patient centered approach is:

Provider:
Let me make sure I explained that clearly. What questions do you have? *(invites dialogue)*

Patient:
I'm scared about what this means.

Provider:
You'll be fine. *(empty reassurance)*

This offers empty reassurance without meeting the fear. A grounded, empathic response is:

Provider:
It's completely understandable to feel scared. I'm here to help you through this. *(grounded reassurance)*

Patient:
Thank you… that helps.

Provider:
We'll take this step by step together. *(reinforces partnership)*

The Illusion of Neutrality

Providers often believe they are speaking objectively, especially when using clinical terminology. However, what is objective in intention is rarely neutral in reception. Words like "negative," "positive," "failure," or "progression" have precise medical meanings, but they also carry emotional associations that patients cannot easily separate.

Telling a patient their test is "negative" may be reassuring in context, but the word itself is inherently loaded. Similarly, describing a treatment as having "failed" can feel like a personal judgment, even if it is meant purely in a clinical sense. Patients may internalize these terms in ways that providers do not anticipate.

The responsibility, then, is not to abandon medical language, but to translate it. To recognize that clarity is not achieved simply by being correct, but by being understood in the way it is intended.

Dialogue: The Illusion of Neutrality (Clinical Words vs. Human Meaning)

Provider:
Your biopsy came back negative.

Patient:
Negative… that sounds bad.

Provider:
No, negative means nothing was found. *(assumes shared understanding)*

This assumes shared medical understanding, which patients often don't have. A clearer, more reassuring alternative is:

Provider:
The biopsy did not show any cancer, which is good news. *(translates meaning clearly)*

Patient:

Oh… okay. I wasn't sure what that meant.

Provider:
The imaging, however, shows some progression. *(technical term without context)*

Patient:
Progression? So, it's getting worse?

Provider:
Yes, the disease has progressed. *(abrupt, emotionally heavy)*

These technical terms land abruptly and can feel emotionally heavy. A softer, more contextual framing is:

Provider:
The condition has changed since your last scan, and we'll need to adjust the plan. *(softer, clearer framing)*

Patient:
Did the treatment fail?

Provider:
Yes, the treatment failed. *(feels like personal defeat)*

Patient:
I did everything I was supposed to…

This wording can feel like a personal defeat. A response that removes blame and restores perspective is:

Provider:
This treatment didn't work as we hoped, and that's not because of anything you did. *(removes blame)*

Patient:
That's a relief to hear…

Provider:
Your results are positive. *(confusing emotional contradiction)*

Patient:
Positive? That sounds good… right?

Provider:
In this case, positive means the condition is present. *(delayed clarification)*

This creates confusion because the emotional meaning of "positive" contradicts the medical meaning. A clearer, immediate explanation is:

Provider:
The test shows that the condition is there, so we can now focus on treating it. *(immediate clarity)*

Patient:
This is a lot to take in.

Provider:
These are standard findings. *(feels minimizing)*

This can feel minimizing, especially when the patient is overwhelmed. A response that respects their experience is:

Provider:
I know this may not feel routine to you, even if we see it often. Let's go through it together. *(respects patient experience)*

Patient:
Thank you for explaining it that way.

Provider:
Of course. I want to make sure what I say is not just accurate, but clear and helpful for you. *(Land: reinforces intention and trust)*

The Weight of Certainty and Uncertainty

Another critical dimension of language lies in how certainty is expressed. Providers are often trained to project confidence. This is important for leadership and decision-making. However, overconfidence in language can create false expectations, while excessive caution can create unnecessary fear. Saying, "This will take care of the problem," may offer reassurance, but it risks eroding trust if outcomes differ. On the other hand, saying, "We're not sure what this is," without context can leave a patient feeling abandoned.

A more balanced approach might sound like: "Based on what we know, this treatment has a strong chance of helping, and we'll monitor closely as we go." This kind of language acknowledges uncertainty without surrendering confidence. It invites the patient into a process rather than presenting medicine as absolute.

Dialogue: The Weight of Certainty and Uncertainty

Provider:
This medication will take care of the problem. *(over certainty)*

Patient:
So, once I take it, I'll be fine?

Provider:
Yes, this should fix it completely. *(unrealistic expectation)*

Patient:
Okay… that makes me feel better.

Patient (later):
It didn't work like you said...

Provider:
Sometimes that happens. *(trust erosion after certainty)*

This erodes trust because earlier statements conveyed absolute certainty. A more grounded alternative is:

Provider:
Based on what we know, this medication has a strong chance of helping. *(grounded confidence)*

Patient:
So, it should work?

Provider:
There's a good likelihood, and we'll keep a close eye on how you respond. *(realistic framing)*

Patient:
That makes sense.

Provider:
We're not sure what this is. *(uncertainty without support)*

Patient:
You don't know? That's scary.

Provider:
We'll need more tests. *(feels incomplete, distant)*

This expresses uncertainty without support or direction. A clearer, more structured alternative is:

Provider:
We don't have a full answer yet, but we do have a clear next step to figure it out. *(structured uncertainty)*

Patient:
Okay... that helps a little.

Provider:
We'll go through this step by step, and I'll keep you informed along the way. *(partnership)*

Patient:
Is this something serious?

Provider:
It could be, or it might not be. *(vague, unanchored uncertainty)*

Patient:
That doesn't make me feel any better...

This is vague and unanchored, which heightens fear. A more calibrated, reassuring alternative is:

Provider:
There are a few possibilities, some more serious than others, but right now nothing suggests an immediate danger. *(calibrated reassurance)*

Patient:
That's reassuring to hear.
Provider:
You'll be fine. *(empty certainty)*

Patient:
I hope so...

This offers empty certainty and can feel dismissive. A more honest and supportive response is:

Provider:
I can't promise exactly how this will unfold, but we have good options and we'll face this together. *(honest confidence)*

Patient:
Thank you... that feels more real.

One of the most overlooked aspects of medical language is how it shapes identity. Referring to someone as "a diabetic," "a smoker," or "a non-compliant patient" reduces a complex human being to a single characteristic. While these labels may be efficient in clinical shorthand, they carry unintended consequences.

Patients hear these labels not as descriptors, but as definitions. They can feel judged, categorized, or diminished. Over time, this can affect how patients see themselves and how they engage with care.

A simple shift—from "a diabetic" to "a patient living with diabetes"—restores personhood. It may seem minor, but it reflects a deeper orientation: seeing the individual before the condition.

The Subtle Harm of Reassurance

Reassurance is a cornerstone of medical communication, yet it can be surprisingly easy to do poorly. Phrases like "Don't worry," "You'll be fine," or "It's nothing serious" are often offered with good intentions. However, they can unintentionally invalidate the patient's feelings. When a patient is worried, telling them not to worry does not remove the concern. It can create distance. The patient may feel misunderstood or dismissed, even if the provider is trying to comfort them.

More effective reassurance acknowledges the emotion first: "I can see why this would worry you. Let's go through what we know and what it means." This approach does not eliminate fear immediately, but it creates a space where fear can be addressed.

Dialogue: The Subtle Harm of Reassurance

Patient:
I've been really worried about these symptoms.

Provider:
Don't worry, it's nothing serious. *(dismisses concern)*

Patient:
...It still feels serious to me.

Provider:
You'll be fine. *(empty reassurance)*

Patient:
I hope so, but I'm still anxious.

Provider:
There's no reason to be upset. *(invalidates emotion)*

Patient:
It just doesn't feel like that to me.

Provider:
It's probably nothing. *(vague, minimizing)*

Patient:
I don't feel any better hearing that.

These responses intend to reassure but instead dismiss, minimize, or invalidate the patient's emotional reality. A more effective approach acknowledges the feeling first and then offers clarity. The same moment can unfold differently when reassurance is grounded in empathy:

Provider:
I can see this has really been worrying you. *(acknowledges emotion)*

Patient:
It has... I haven't been able to stop thinking about it.

Provider:
That makes sense. When something feels unfamiliar, it's easy for your mind to go to worst-case scenarios. *(normalizes feeling)*

Patient:
Exactly.

Provider:
Let's go through what we know so far and what it likely means. *(creates structure)*

Patient:
Okay, that would help.

Provider:
From what you've described, there's nothing immediately dangerous. *(grounded reassurance)*

Patient:
That's good to hear.

Provider:
At the same time, your concern is valid, and we'll take it seriously. *(validates + reassures)*

Patient:
I appreciate that.

Patient:
So, I'm not overreacting?

Provider:
Not at all. Anyone in your position would feel this way. *(removes self-doubt)*

Patient:
That makes me feel better.

Provider:
We'll take this step by step, and I'll be here to guide you through it. *(supportive presence)*

Patient:
Thank you… that actually calms me down.

Timing and Delivery

Words do not exist in isolation. Their impact is shaped by when and how they are delivered. A technically correct explanation given too quickly, or without pause, can overwhelm. Important information can be lost not because it was unclear, but because it was poorly timed.

Patients need space to process. Silence, often uncomfortable for clinicians, plays an essential role here. It allows words to settle. It gives patients the opportunity to react, to ask, to absorb.

Similarly, the sequencing of information matters. Leading with the most alarming detail without context can heighten anxiety unnecessarily. Building a narrative—starting with orientation, then moving into specifics—helps patients follow and understand.

Dialogue: Timing and Delivery

Provider:
Your scan shows a mass, and we're concerned it could be malignant, so we'll need more imaging and possibly a biopsy. *(overwhelming, no pause)*

Patient:
Wait… a mass? Malignant? I'm not following…

Provider:
It means there's something there that could be serious. *(abrupt clarification)*

Patient:
This is a lot… I didn't expect this.

Provider:
We need to move quickly on this. *(escalates anxiety)*

Patient:
I feel like I can't even think right now.

Provider:
Do you have any questions? *(poorly timed invitation)*

Patient:
I don't even know what to ask…

This sequence is medically accurate but delivered too quickly, without pacing, structure, or space for the patient to process. The result is overwhelm rather than clarity. The same information can land very differently when it is slowed down, sequenced, and supported:

Provider:
I want to go over your scan results with you, and we can take it one step at a time. *(sets structure)*

Patient:
Okay…

Provider:
The scan shows an area that we didn't expect to see. *(gentle entry)*

Patient:
What does that mean?

Provider:
It means there's something there we need to understand better. *(controlled pacing)*
(brief pause)

Patient:
…Is it something serious?

Provider:
It could be, but we don't know yet. The next step is to get more information so we can be certain.
(balanced clarity)

Patient:
Okay… I think I'm following.

Provider:
I know this may feel overwhelming. We can pause here for a moment if you need. *(allows processing)*

Patient:
I appreciate that…

Provider:
When you're ready, I can explain what the next steps look like and what each one involves. *(paced sequencing)*

Patient:
Yes, please.

Provider:
We'll start with additional imaging, and depending on that, we may consider a biopsy to get a clear answer. *(structured explanation)*

Patient:
That makes more sense now.

Provider:
And as we go through this, please stop me anytime if something isn't clear. *(keeps space open)*

Patient:
Thank you… that helps me stay grounded.

Micro-Moments That Shape Trust

Trust is not built in grand gestures. It is built in small, repeated moments. A provider who says, "Let me make sure I explained that clearly," signals humility and care. One who says, "Do you understand?" may unintentionally sound impatient or evaluative. The difference lies not in intent, but in perception. Even subtle shifts—using "we" instead of "you," or "let's look at this together" instead of "here's what you need to do"—can transform the dynamic from directive to collaborative. Patients are more likely to engage when they feel included rather than instructed.

Dialogue: Micro-Moments That Shape Trust

Provider:
You need to take this medication twice a day. *(directive, impersonal)*

Patient:
Okay…

Provider:
Do you understand? *(evaluative tone)*

Patient:
I think so…

Provider:
Just follow the instructions and you'll be fine. *(dismissive, closed)*

Patient:
Alright…

These responses are directive, evaluative, and closed. They place the patient in a passive role and can create distance or self-doubt. The same moments can build trust when the language shifts toward collaboration, clarity, and shared ownership:

Provider:
Let's go over how we'll approach this together. *(collaborative tone)*

Patient:
Okay, I like that.

Provider:
We'll start this medication twice daily, and we can adjust as needed. *(flexible partnership)*

Patient:
That sounds manageable.

Provider:
Let me make sure I explained that clearly. What questions do you have? *(invites dialogue)*

Patient:
Actually, what if I miss a dose?

Provider:
That's a great question. If that happens, we can talk through what to do so it doesn't feel stressful. *(supportive response)*

Patient:
I appreciate that.

Provider:
You need to change your diet. *(directive, isolating)*

Patient:
I've tried before… it's hard.

Provider:
Well, you have to try harder. *(judgmental)*

Patient:
...That's discouraging.

This exchange becomes judgmental and isolating, making the patient feel solely responsible for success or failure. A collaborative reframing shifts ownership to a shared effort:

Provider:
Let's look at your diet together and see what small changes feel realistic. *(shared ownership)*

Patient:
That feels more doable.

Provider:
We don't have to change everything at once. We can start with one step. *(reduces pressure)*

Patient:
I think I can do that.

Provider:
Here's what you need to do next. *(authoritative)*

Patient:
Okay...

This phrasing is authoritative and one directional. A more inclusive approach keeps the patient engaged and supported:

Provider:
Here are the next steps, and we'll go through them together, so nothing feels unclear. *(inclusive guidance)*

Patient:
Thank you... that makes me feel more involved.

The Risk of Habitual Language

Over time, providers develop patterns of speech. Certain phrases become automatic, repeated across encounters. While this increases efficiency, it can also lead to disconnection. Language becomes standardized, but patients are not.

What feels routine to the provider can feel impersonal to the patient. This is particularly true in difficult conversations, where patients are highly sensitive to tone and wording. Revisiting one's own language is therefore not an academic exercise. It is a practical necessity. It requires awareness, reflection, and a willingness to adjust.

Dialogue: The Risk of Habitual Language

Provider:
This is a very common condition. *(automatic, impersonal)*

Patient:
It doesn't feel common to me…

Provider:
We see this all the time. *(routine language, distancing)*

Patient:
I guess… but it's new for me.

Provider:
You'll just need to follow the standard protocol. *(scripted, non-individualized)*

Patient:
That sounds… kind of generic.

Provider:
That's what we usually do. *(reinforces routine over person)*

Patient:
I was hoping for something more specific to me.

These responses rely on routine, scripted language. They may be efficient for the provider but can feel impersonal or minimizing to the patient. A more intentional approach personalizes the moment and restores connection:

Provider:
I realize this may be something we see often, but for you, this is a new and important experience. *(personalizes care)*

Patient:
Yes, exactly.

Provider:
Let's talk about how this is affecting you specifically. *(shifts focus to individual)*

Patient:
I appreciate that.

Provider:
There are standard approaches we use, but we can tailor them to fit your situation. *(flexible, patient-centered)*

Patient:
That makes me feel more comfortable.

Provider:
You'll be fine, this happens all the time. *(habitual reassurance)*

Patient:
It still feels serious to me.

Provider:
There's nothing unusual here. *(minimizes uniqueness)*

Patient:
I don't feel heard.

This habitual reassurance minimizes the patient's lived experience and reinforces the sense of being "just another case." A more mindful shift acknowledges individuality and reopens trust:

Provider:
Even if this is something we treat regularly, I want to understand how it's impacting you personally. *(restores connection)*

Patient:
Thank you… that means a lot.

Provider:
I'm going to slow down for a moment and make sure I'm not just repeating what I usually say. *(self-awareness)*

Patient:
I can tell the difference.

Provider:
You're not just another case. Let's make sure this plan truly fits you. *(individualized care)*

Patient:
That helps me trust this process much more.

For Healthcare Students: Building Awareness Early

Students often focus on learning what to say. Equally important is learning how words are received. This requires observation, feedback, and practice. It involves noticing not just outcomes, but reactions. How does the patient respond when certain phrases are used? Do they lean in or withdraw? Do they ask more questions or become quiet? These cues are invaluable. They provide real-time feedback on the impact of language.

Dialogue: For Healthcare Students — Building Awareness Early

Medical Student:
Your labs are normal, so there's nothing to worry about. *(dismissive phrasing)*

Patient:
...I still don't feel right.

Medical Student:
Everything looks fine medically. *(repeats data, misses reaction)*

Patient:
Okay...

(Patient becomes quieter, avoids eye contact)

Attending (later):
What did you notice when you said that?

Medical Student:
I gave correct information... but they seemed to shut down.

Attending:
Exactly. You were accurate but not attuned to how it landed.

This sequence shows how technically correct statements can still miss the patient's emotional reality. Building awareness early means noticing reactions, not just delivering information. When the student re-approaches with attention to tone and response, the interaction shifts:

Medical Student (re-approaching):
Your labs came back within the normal range. *(clear but neutral)*

Patient:
That's good, I guess...

Medical Student:
I notice you seem unsure—can you tell me what still feels concerning? *(observes reaction)*

Patient:
I still feel the symptoms, and it's worrying me.

Medical Student:
That makes sense. Even with normal results, your experience is still real. *(validates)*

Patient:
Yes, exactly.

Attending (after visit):

What did you see change?

Medical Student:
The patient opened up more the second time.

Attending:
Why do you think that happened?

Medical Student:
I paid attention to their reaction, not just the results.

Attending:
That's the key. Words are not just spoken—they are received.

Medical Student:
So, I should watch how patients respond in real time?

Attending:
Yes. Do they lean in, ask questions, relax—or do they withdraw?

Medical Student:
I see... it's not just what I say, but how it affects them.

Attending:
Exactly. That awareness is what turns communication into care.

Medical Student:
I'll start paying closer attention to those moments.

Attending:
Good. That's where your real learning begins.

For Experienced Providers: Refinement, Not Reinvention

For those with years of practice, the goal is not to overhaul communication, but to refine it. Small adjustments can yield significant changes. Replacing a single phrase, adding a moment of acknowledgment, or pausing before responding can shift the entire tone of an interaction. This is not about perfection. It is about awareness.

Dialogue: For Experienced Providers — Refinement, Not Reinvention

Provider:
This is straightforward. We'll start treatment today. *(Harm: efficient but abrupt)*

Patient:
Okay... that feels fast.

Provider:
It's the standard approach. *(Harm: routine, not personalized)*

Patient:
I guess…

(Provider pauses, notices hesitation)

These responses are efficient but can feel abrupt or impersonal. Even experienced clinicians benefit from slowing down, noticing cues, and adjusting in real time. A small shift in pacing or acknowledgment can change the entire tone of the encounter:

Provider:
Let me slow down for a moment. I may have gone through that quickly. *(self-awareness)*

Patient:
I appreciate that.

Provider:
While this is a common approach, I want to make sure it feels right for you. *(personalization)*

Patient:
That helps me feel more comfortable.

Patient:
I'm just trying to process everything.

Provider:
It's a lot of information. *(generic acknowledgment)*

Patient:
Yeah…

This acknowledgment is technically correct but generic. A more attuned response names what the clinician is actually observing:

Provider:
I can see this is a lot to take in right now. *(more specific attunement)*

Patient:
It really is.

Provider:
You'll need to follow this plan closely. *(directive tone)*

Patient:
I'll try.

This directive tone can feel onesided. A collaborative adjustment helps the plan feel more achievable:

Provider:
Let's go through the plan together and see how it fits into your daily life. *(collaborative adjustment)*

Patient:
That makes it feel more manageable.

Patient:
What if this doesn't work?

Provider:
We'll deal with that if it happens. *(dismissive uncertainty)*

Patient:
That's a little unsettling…

This response leaves uncertainty uncontained. A more structured reassurance helps the patient feel supported rather than dismissed:

Provider:
That's a fair question. If this approach doesn't give us the results we want, we have other options we can move to. *(reassuring structure)*

Patient:
That helps me feel less stuck.

Provider:
Any questions? *(closed, routine)*

Patient:
Not sure…

This routine closing can feel perfunctory. A more open invitation encourages real dialogue:

Provider:
I want to make sure I explained things clearly—what's on your mind right now? *(open, inviting)*

Patient:
Actually, I do have a few questions.

Provider:
Good. Let's take them one at a time. *(calm, present guidance)*

Patient:
Thank you… I feel more at ease now.

Language as a Clinical Tool

When used thoughtfully, language becomes more than communication. It becomes a tool for care. It can reduce anxiety, clarify understanding, and strengthen the therapeutic relationship. When used without awareness, it can do the opposite. It can create confusion, distance, and unintended harm. The difference often lies in details that are easy to overlook.

Dialogue: Language as a Clinical Tool

Provider:
Your condition is stable. *(technically correct but vague)*

Patient:
I'm not sure what that means… is that good or bad?

Provider:
It means it's not changing. *(still unclear emotionally)*

Patient:
I still feel uncertain.

This explanation is medically accurate but emotionally vague. A clearer, more contextualized framing helps the patient understand what "stable" actually means:

Provider:
What I'm seeing is that your condition hasn't worsened, which is a positive sign. *(clearer meaning)*

Patient:
That makes me feel a bit better.

Patient:
I've been really anxious about all of this.

Provider:
That's understandable. *(generic, limited impact)*

This acknowledgment is technically correct but too general to land. A more specific reflection shows the provider is truly hearing the patient:

Provider:
I can hear how much this has been weighing on you day to day. *(specific acknowledgment)*

Patient:
Yes, exactly.

Provider:
Just take the medication and come back in a month. *(transactional)*

Patient:
Okay…

This phrasing is transactional and leaves the patient alone with the plan. A supportive, practical framing helps the patient feel guided rather than dismissed:

Provider:
Let's talk about how this medication fits into your routine, so it feels manageable between now and our next visit. *(supportive planning)*

Patient:
That helps me think about it more clearly.

Patient:
What should I expect?

Provider:
Side effects are possible. *(vague, anxiety-provoking)*

Patient:
Like what?

This answer is vague and can heighten anxiety. A more specific and supportive explanation helps the patient feel prepared rather than worried:

Provider:
Some people notice mild fatigue or nausea, but many tolerate it well. If anything concerns you, I want you to reach out. *(specific + supportive)*

Patient:
That makes me feel more prepared.

Provider:
We'll monitor this. *(distant, undefined)*

Patient:
What does that involve?

This reassurance is too undefined to be comforting. A clearer description of the process helps the patient feel held rather than left in the dark:

Provider:
We'll check in regularly and repeat testing if needed, so we can adjust quickly if anything changes. *(clear process)*

Patient:
I like knowing there's a plan.

Provider:
Okay, that's it for today. *(abrupt close)*

This closing is abrupt and can leave the patient feeling unfinished. A more thoughtful ending ensures clarity and emotional closure:

Provider:
Before we finish, I want to make sure you feel clear and supported—what questions or concerns are still on your mind? *(thoughtful closure)*

Conclusion: The Responsibility of Words

Every conversation in medicine carries weight. Not because every word must be perfect, but because every word contributes to an experience the patient will carry forward. Patients may forget the specifics of what was said. They may not recall the exact terminology or sequence of explanations. But they will remember how the words felt. They will remember whether they felt seen, respected, and supported. Words that land do more than inform. They connect. Words that harm rarely do so through intention. They do so through absence—absence of awareness, of presence, of consideration for how language is received. The opportunity, then, is not to speak more, but to speak more thoughtfully. Because in medicine, language is never just language; it is care, delivered in real time.

Chapter 8

The 10-Minute Rule — Creating Meaningful Connections Even in Limited Time

One of the most persistent myths in medicine is that meaningful connection requires long conversations. It does not. What it requires is *undivided presence.* Ten minutes, when used deliberately, can carry more emotional weight and clinical impact than thirty minutes of distracted care.

The patient does not measure time the way a provider does. They measure *attention.* They measure whether you saw them, whether you heard them, and whether you understood them. In those first moments, before a word of diagnosis is processed, the foundation of trust is either built or weakened.

The 10-minute rule is not about compressing care. It is about *structuring presence.*

The first minute is decisive. When you enter the room, pause. Sit if possible. Make eye contact before looking at a chart or screen. Your body language communicates immediately whether the patient is a priority or an interruption. A rushed entrance creates distance that is difficult to recover from, no matter how skilled the explanation that follows.

The next three minutes should belong entirely to the patient. Let them speak without interruption. Most patients complete their primary concern in under two minutes if allowed to do so. Interrupting early may save seconds, but it costs understanding. More importantly, it signals that efficiency matters more than their experience.

The middle phase is where competence and connection merge. Ask focused questions, but do not lose the human thread. A simple acknowledgment such as, "That sounds frustrating," or "I can see why that concerns you," does not slow the visit. It anchors it. Patients are far more receptive to medical reasoning when they feel emotionally recognized.

The final minutes are where clarity is secured. Summarize what you have heard. Outline the plan in clear, simple terms. Then pause again and ask, "What questions do you have?" This subtle shift—from *Do you have questions?* to *What questions do you have?*—assumes engagement rather than dismissing it. It invites participation.

What makes this rule powerful is not its structure alone, but its intention. You are not trying to *appear* present. You are choosing to *be* present within the constraints that modern medicine imposes. Patients rarely say, "My doctor didn't spend enough time explaining the pharmacology." They say, "My doctor didn't listen," or "I felt rushed," or "I didn't feel like I mattered." Those impressions are not determined by the clock. They are determined by how the minutes are used.

The provider who masters the 10-minute rule understands something essential: Connection is not a luxury added to care. It is a force that shapes how care is received, remembered, and followed. In limited time, presence becomes more—not less—important.

The 10-Minute Rule in Practice — A Complete Clinical Scenario

The purpose of this demonstration is not to show perfection, but to make visible what *intentional presence* looks like when time is limited.

Minute 0: The Entrance

Dr. Patel pauses briefly outside the door, hand on the handle. A breath. A reset. Then she enters.

Dr. Patel (sitting down, not standing)**:**
Good morning, Mr. Lewis. I'm Dr. Patel.

(She makes eye contact before opening the chart. Her posture is relaxed, slightly leaning forward.)

Patient:
Morning.

Dr. Patel:
It's good to meet you.

(A brief pause. No typing. No rushing.)

Minutes 1–3: The Patient Speaks

Dr. Patel:
What brought you in today?

(She remains silent. Attentive. No interruptions.)

Patient:
I've been having this chest discomfort… not really pain, more like pressure. It started a couple of weeks ago. At first I ignored it, but it's been happening more often. Especially when I walk upstairs.

And… I don't know… I guess I got a little worried.

(He glances down.)

I didn't want to overreact, but my wife insisted I come in.

(He stops.)

Dr. Patel (after a brief pause):
I'm really glad you came in.

(She lets that land before continuing.)

Minutes 3–6: Clinical Focus Without Losing Connection

Dr. Patel:
Can you tell me more about the pressure? Where exactly do you feel it?

(The questioning becomes structured, but her tone remains calm and human.)

Patient:
Right here. Center of my chest. Sometimes it moves a little to the left.

Dr. Patel:
Does it come on with activity every time, or only sometimes?

(They move through key diagnostic questions: duration, radiation, associated symptoms.)

Patient:
Sometimes I feel a little short of breath too. That's what's been bothering me.

(His voice tightens slightly.)

Dr. Patel (gently):
That sounds unsettling.

(She does not overreact. She does not dismiss. She acknowledges.)

Minutes 6–8: Integration and Meaning

Dr. Patel:
Let me make sure I understand this clearly.

(She turns slightly toward him, summarizing.)

You've been having a pressure-like feeling in the center of your chest for about two weeks. It happens more with activity, like climbing stairs, and sometimes comes with shortness of breath. And it's been becoming more frequent. Is that right?

Patient:
Yes… exactly.

(There is visible relief in being accurately understood.)

Dr. Patel:
Given what you're describing, this is something we need to take seriously and evaluate carefully. There are a few possible causes, and some of them involve the heart, so we don't want to ignore it.

(Her tone is steady. Clear. Not alarmist, but not minimizing.)

Minutes 8–10: Clarity, Partnership, and Closure

Dr. Patel:
Here's what I'd like to do next.

(She outlines the plan in simple, structured language.)

We'll start with an EKG today and some blood work. I'd also like to arrange a stress test to see how your heart is functioning during activity. Based on those results, we'll decide the next steps together.

(She pauses.)

I also want you to know—you did the right thing coming in.

(Another pause.)

What questions do you have?

Patient (after a moment):
Do you think this is… something serious?

Dr. Patel:
It *could be*, which is why we're going to evaluate it thoroughly. But the important thing is—we're addressing it now, and we'll move step by step with you.

(She maintains eye contact. No typing yet.)

Patient:
Okay… that makes me feel better.

Final Moment: The Exit

(Dr. Patel stands but does not rush away.)

Dr. Patel:
We'll get started on those tests right away. I'll be with you through this process.

(A slight nod. A final moment of acknowledgment. Then she exits.)

Why This Works

Nothing in this interaction required more time than a typical visit. What made it different was not duration, but *design*:

- The patient was allowed to speak without interruption.
- The provider acknowledged emotion without losing clinical focus.
- Information was summarized, not scattered.
- The plan was clear and collaborative.
- The patient left not only informed—but *seen*.

This is the essence of the 10-minute rule: not efficiency alone, not empathy alone, but the deliberate integration of both within the time that already exists.

Part III

Navigating Difficult Clinical Scenarios

Chapter 9 Delivering Bad News 104

Chapter 10 When the Diagnosis Is Uncertain 127

Chapter 11 Managing Patient Anxiety and Fear 136

Chapter 12 The Angry or Distrustful Patient 158

Chapter 13 End-of-Life Conversations 175

Chapter 9

Delivering Bad News

Clarity, Pacing, and Emotional Awareness

There are moments in medicine when knowledge alone is not enough. Delivering bad news is one of them. In these moments, the provider is not only a source of information but a stabilizing presence in the face of uncertainty, fear, and often life-altering reality. What patients remember is not only *what* was said, but *how* it was said, *when* it was said, and *whether they felt alone while hearing it.*

Bad news is not a single statement. It is a process.

The First Responsibility: Prepare the Space

Before a word is spoken, the environment must be intentional. Sit down. Eliminate distractions. Silence the computer or at least turn your body fully toward the patient. If possible, ensure privacy. These small adjustments communicate something profound: *this moment matters.*

Rushing into difficult news while standing at the door, hand on the handle, signals discomfort and avoidance. Patients feel that immediately.

The Pre-Encounter Briefing

Dr. Reynolds (speaking calmly to his medical assistant outside the room):
Before I go in, I want to make sure the room is set up properly. This is not a routine visit.

(He pauses to ensure attention.)

First, no interruptions. Please hold any non-urgent calls and let the front desk know I'm not to be pulled out unless it's critical.

Second, I don't want the patient sitting on the exam table if we can avoid it. Have them seated in a chair or lower the table so we're at eye level. This needs to feel like a conversation, not an exam.

Third, make sure the room is quiet. Turn off anything unnecessary. If the TV is on, it should be off. If there's noise in the hallway, close the door fully.

Inside the Room: Final Adjustments

(The assistant enters the room briefly before the provider.)

Assistant (to patient, gently):
Dr. Reynolds will be in shortly. Before he comes in, I just want to make sure you're comfortable.

(She adjusts the chair slightly so it faces where the doctor will sit, not angled away. She places a box of tissues within reach, but not in a way that feels presumptive.)

Is there anyone you'd like to have with you right now? We can bring them in if you'd like.

(She gives the patient a moment to respond.)

Coordination with the Provider

(Assistant steps out and quietly updates Dr. Reynolds.)

Assistant:
They're alone right now, but I asked if they wanted someone with them. The room is set, the door is closed, and there shouldn't be any interruptions.

Dr. Reynolds (nodding):
Thank you. That's exactly what we need.

The Subtle but Critical Details

Before the provider enters:

- The computer screen is either turned away or dimmed.
- The provider's chair is positioned close enough for conversation, not distance.
- The physical barrier between doctor and patient (desk, equipment) is minimized.
- The patient is not left exposed in a gown if it can be avoided.

None of these steps take more than a minute. But together, they transform the emotional tone of the room.

Teaching the Why

(Later, with a trainee observing)

Dr. Reynolds:
If the environment feels rushed, distracted, or clinical, the patient senses that before we say a single word. They may not be able to explain it—but they feel it.

When we prepare the space properly, we are telling them something without speaking: *You matter. This moment matters. I am here with you.*

What This Achieves

By the time the provider walks into the room:

- The patient is not bracing for a rushed interaction
- The environment supports stillness, not distraction
- The provider is free to focus entirely on the conversation

This is not about theatrics; it is about alignment. The team, the space, and the provider are all communicating the same message—before a single word of bad news is delivered.

Start with Awareness, Not Assumption

Before delivering information, understand what the patient already knows:

- "What have you been told so far?"
- "What is your sense of what might be going on?"

This does two things. It prevents overwhelming the patient with information they are not prepared for, and it reveals emotional readiness. Some patients are already anticipating the worst. Others are not. Your delivery must meet them where they are, not where you are.

Dr. Alvarez (sitting down, calm, steady):
Hi, Mr. Carter. Thank you for waiting.

(He makes eye contact. No chart in hand yet. No computer use.)

Patient:
Of course.

(A brief pause. The provider does not rush forward.)

Dr. Alvarez:
Before we go over the results, I'd like to understand what you've been told so far.

(The tone is neutral. Not leading. Not alarming.)

Patient (exhales slightly):
Well… they said the scan showed something on my lung. A mass, I think they called it.

(He watches the doctor carefully.)

Dr. Alvarez (nods):
Okay.

(He allows space, signaling there is more the patient can say.)

Patient:
They didn't really explain much. Just that I needed to follow up here.

(Pause.)

I mean… I've been trying not to think the worst, but… you hear things.

The Second Awareness Question

Dr. Alvarez (gently):
When you say 'the worst,' what's been on your mind?

(This question is precise. It invites the patient to define their own fear.)

Patient (hesitates, then quietly):
Cancer.

(The word lands heavily in the room.)

The Provider Reads Readiness

At this point, the provider has learned something critical:

- The patient already suspects a serious diagnosis
- The emotional ground has already shifted
- The word *cancer* has already been spoken by the patient, not introduced abruptly by the provider

This changes everything about how the next sentence will be received.

Meeting the Patient Where They Are

Dr. Alvarez (steady, direct, but not abrupt):
I understand why that would be on your mind.

(A pause. Then, clearly.)

The results do show a mass in your lung, and we are concerned that this could be cancer.

(He does not rush past the statement.)

Why This Approach Matters

Because the provider began with awareness:

- The patient was not blindsided
- The language matched the patient's own level of concern
- The emotional transition was *continuous*, not abrupt

Had the patient instead said, "I was told it's probably nothing," the provider's approach would shift—slowing down further, preparing the patient more gradually before naming the diagnosis.

The Subtle Skill Being Demonstrated

The provider is not simply gathering information. He is calibrating the conversation. He is answering an unspoken question: *How much truth can this patient absorb right now, and how should it be delivered?*

The Teaching Point

Starting with awareness is not a formality. It is a diagnostic step—just as important as any lab result. Because if you deliver the right information at the wrong emotional moment, it will not be heard. But if you meet the patient where they already are, the same words can be understood, processed, and remembered. And in that moment, understanding is everything.

The Moment of Clarity

When it is time to speak, clarity matters more than eloquence. Avoid euphemisms. Avoid vague language that forces the patient to interpret meaning under stress. Statements like *"It doesn't look good"* or *"We found something concerning"* create confusion and prolong anxiety.

Instead, speak plainly: "The results show that you have cancer," or "The scan shows that the disease has spread." Then stop. Silence is not a failure of communication. It is an essential part of it. The patient needs a moment to process what was just said. Filling that silence too quickly is often a way to relieve the provider's discomfort, not the patient's.

A Dialogue Demonstration

The room has already been prepared. The patient has spoken. The provider understands what the patient knows and fears. Now comes the moment that cannot be softened, only delivered well.

Dr. Bennett (sitting, steady, no computer, full eye contact):
Mr. Harris… I have the results of your biopsy.

(A brief pause. Not long, but intentional.)

Patient (quietly):
Okay…

(He braces slightly. His hands tighten.)

The Statement

Dr. Bennett (clear, direct, calm):
The results show that you have cancer.

(Silence.)

There is no immediate explanation, no rapid follow-up, no attempt to cushion or reinterpret—just presence.)

(The room becomes still. The patient looks down. Several seconds pass. He exhales slowly, almost as if the air has been taken out of him.)

Patient (barely above a whisper):
…Okay.

(Another pause. His eyes begin to well slightly, but he does not fully cry.)

The Provider Holds the Space

Dr. Bennett does not interrupt the silence or rush to explain staging, treatment, or statistics. He simply watches and waits, because this moment does not belong to the provider—it belongs to the patient.

The First Response

Patient (after several seconds):
What… what kind?

(Now the patient is ready for more.)

The Next Layer

Dr. Bennett (still calm, still measured):
It is a type of lung cancer called non-small cell lung cancer.

(He pauses again, allowing the words to land in smaller, manageable pieces.)

Why This Works

If Dr. Bennett had said, "We found something concerning, and it doesn't look good, and we're worried it might be cancer, and we'll need to do more tests," the patient would be left in uncertainty, trying to decode meaning under stress. Instead, clarity removes the burden of interpretation.

The Discipline of Restraint

The most difficult part of this moment is not saying the words, it is what comes after. The instinct to fill the silence is strong:

- To explain immediately
- To reassure prematurely
- To soften what feels unbearable

But when providers speak too quickly after delivering bad news, they often do so to relieve *their own* discomfort. Silence, in contrast, serves the patient. It gives:

- Space to absorb
- Space to react
- Space to begin forming questions

The Teaching Point

Clarity is not cruelty, and silence is not abandonment. When done correctly, they are forms of respect. You are not leaving the patient alone in that silence. You are staying with them in it. And in that brief, quiet space, the reality has a chance to be understood—not just heard.

Read the Emotional Response

There is no single correct reaction to bad news. Some patients cry. Some ask immediate questions. Some become silent. Some appear unaffected. Your role is not to control the reaction, but to *recognize and respond to it*:

- "I can see this is a lot to take in."
- "It's okay to feel overwhelmed."
- "We can go through this step by step."

These statements do not fix the situation. They anchor the patient within it.

Reading and Responding to Emotion

What Happens Immediately After the Words Land

The moment after clarity is not empty. It is filled with reaction, often unstructured and unpredictable. This is where many providers, even highly skilled ones, lose connection. Not because they lack empathy, but because they move too quickly back into information.

What follows is not about controlling emotion. It is about recognizing it, allowing it, and responding to it without losing presence.

A Dialogue Demonstration

(The diagnosis has just been delivered.)

Dr. Bennett (quiet, present):
The results show that you have cancer.

(Silence follows. The provider remains still.)

Patient (staring down, voice tight):
...I... I don't even know what to say.

(His breathing becomes shallow. His hands begin to tremble slightly.)

The Provider Names What Is Seen

Dr. Bennett (gently):
I can see this is a lot to take in.

(He does not interpret beyond what is visible. He does not assume specific feelings like fear or anger. He reflects what is observable.)

Patient (voice breaking slightly):
Yeah... I just... I wasn't expecting this.

The Provider Validates Without Taking Over

Dr. Bennett:
That makes sense.

(A brief pause.)

Most people aren't prepared to hear something like this.

Allowing the Reaction to unfold

(The patient leans forward, elbows on knees, hands covering part of his face.)

Patient:
What does this mean… am I…?

(He cannot finish the sentence.)

The Provider Responds to the Emotion First, Not the Question

Dr. Bennett (soft, steady):
We're going to take this one step at a time.

(He does not immediately jump into prognosis or statistics.)

You don't have to figure everything out right now.

Why This Matters

In moments like this, patients are not yet asking clinical questions. They are expressing emotional overload *through* questions.

If the provider answers only the surface question, they miss the deeper need.

A Different Reaction: Anger

Not all responses are quiet.

Patient (suddenly frustrated):
How did this even happen? I just had a check-up last year. Nobody saw anything!

Dr. Bennett (calm, not defensive):
I hear how frustrating that feels.

(Pause.)

Let's go through that together.

A Different Reaction: Silence

Sometimes the patient says nothing at all.

(The patient sits completely still, expression blank.)

Dr. Bennett (after a few seconds):
I'm here with you.

(No pressure to speak. No forced questions.)

The Core Principle

You are not trying to fix the emotion. You are trying to *stabilize the patient within it.* This is done by:

- Noticing what is happening
- Naming it simply
- Allowing space for it
- Responding without rushing past it

What the Patient Experiences

In these moments, the patient is asking—often without words:

- "Is it okay for me to feel this way?"
- "Am I alone in this?"
- "Is this doctor going to stay with me, or move on?"

Your response answers those questions more than any medical explanation can.

The Teaching Point

Emotional awareness is not separate from clinical skill. It is part of it. Because if the patient is overwhelmed, they cannot process what comes next. But if they feel recognized—even briefly—they regain enough stability to continue. And that is what makes the rest of the conversation possible.

Pacing the Information

In moments of distress, cognitive processing narrows. Patients cannot absorb complex explanations all at once. Deliver information in layers:

1. The core reality
2. A brief explanation
3. The immediate next step

Not everything needs to be said at once. In fact, saying too much too quickly often results in the patient retaining very little.

Pacing the Information: A Dialogue Demonstration

The diagnosis has been delivered. The patient has reacted. The emotional ground is still unsteady. This is the moment where many providers make an understandable mistake: they try to explain *everything*. But distress narrows cognition. The patient is not ready for complexity. They are ready for *structure*.

The Setup

Dr. Shah (calm, measured):
The results show that you have colon cancer.

(Silence. The patient absorbs this. A few seconds pass.)

Patient (quietly):
...Okay.

Layer One: The Core Reality

This is not repeated in different words. It is not softened or expanded. It has already been stated clearly. Now, the provider moves forward carefully.

Layer Two: A Brief Explanation

Dr. Shah (after a pause):
This type of cancer starts in the lining of the colon. In your case, we found it during the colonoscopy and confirmed it with a biopsy.

(He stops again. No additional detail yet. No staging, no statistics.)

Patient:
So... it's definitely cancer?

Dr. Shah:
Yes.

(Clear. Direct. No added complexity.)

Layer Three: The Immediate Next Step

Dr. Shah:
The next step is to get a CT scan. That will help us understand whether it's contained or if it has spread. That information guides how we treat it.

(Again, he stops.)

Patient:
Is this… treatable?

The Provider Resists Overloading

This is the moment where the provider *could* explain surgery, chemotherapy regimens, survival rates, and timelines. But instead, he stays within the patient's capacity.

Dr. Shah (stead):
Yes, there are effective treatments. The exact plan depends on what we see on the scan.

(Pause.)

We'll go step by step.

What Was *Not* Said (Intentionally)

The provider did not:

- Launch into a full oncology lecture
- Provide survival statistics prematurely
- Outline every possible treatment pathway
- Fill silence with excessive reassurance

Because doing so would overwhelm rather than inform.

The Rhythm of Pacing

Notice the pattern:

- A statement
- A pause
- A response
- Another pause

This rhythm is not accidental. It creates space for the patient to:

- Process
- Ask
- Regain footing

A Contrast: What Overloading Looks Like

Imagine instead: "This is colon cancer; it's an adenocarcinoma. We'll need staging scans, possibly surgery, maybe chemotherapy depending on lymph node involvement. Survival rates vary, but..."

Within seconds, the patient loses the thread. Not because they are incapable—but because they are overwhelmed.

Returning to the Patient

Dr. Shah (gently):
What questions are coming up for you right now?

Patient (after thinking):
I think... I just need to understand what happens next.

Dr. Shah:
That's exactly where we'll focus.

The Teaching Point

Pacing is not about withholding information; it is about *sequencing it*. You are not delivering less; you are delivering it in a way that can actually be received.

The Principle to Remember

In moments of distress:

- The patient cannot absorb everything
- But they can absorb the *next step*

If they leave understanding only two things—what this is and what happens next—then you have succeeded. Everything else can follow, and it will be better understood because you did not rush it.

Maintain Direction Without Removing Hope

Honesty and hope are not opposites. Hope does not always mean a cure. It may mean time. It may mean comfort. It may mean control over what comes next:

- "We have treatments that we can start."
- "There are options, and we will go through them together."
- "We will focus on what we can do from here."

The patient should never feel abandoned within the truth. The diagnosis has been delivered. The patient understands the seriousness. Emotion has been acknowledged. Information has been paced.

Now comes a critical transition. If the provider stops here, the patient is left in a void. If the provider overreaches with unrealistic reassurance, trust is weakened. This moment requires something more precise: direction anchored in honesty, without removing hope.

The Scenario

Dr. Klein (steady, grounded):
The scan shows that the cancer has spread beyond the original area.

(Silence. The patient absorbs this.)

Patient (quiet, strained):
So... what does that mean?

The Risk in This Moment

The patient is not only asking for information. They are asking: "Is there anything left to hold on to?"

The Provider Provides Direction First Then Introduces Grounded Hope

Dr. Klein:
It means that we are not looking at a simple surgery to remove it. *(Clear. Honest. No evasion.)*

Dr. Klein (continues, calm):
But we do have treatments that we can start.

(Pause. Let that land.)

Patient (looking up slightly):
...You do?

Expanding Hope Without Overpromising

Dr. Klein:
Yes. There are options available—treatments that can slow the disease and help you feel better.

(He does not say "cure" if it is not realistic.)

We'll go through those options together and decide what makes the most sense for you.

The Patient Searches for Meaning

Patient:
So... this isn't the end?

The Provider Grounds the Conversation

Dr. Klein (measured, present):
This is something serious. But there is still a path forward.

(A pause.)

We're going to focus on what we can do from here.

What Just Happened

The provider did not:

- Offer false reassurance
- Avoid the seriousness
- Leave the patient in uncertainty

Instead, he did something more difficult. He held two truths at the same time:

- The situation is serious
- There are still meaningful actions to take

A More Fragile Scenario

Sometimes hope must shift even further.

Patient (voice shaking):
Am I dying?

Dr. Klein (quiet, direct):
This is a life-threatening illness.

(Pause. Then gently.)

But right now, our focus is on treating it and supporting you through this.

The Nature of Hope in Medicine

Hope is not always about survival. It can be about:

- Time
- Symptom relief
- Meaningful decisions
- Not being alone

Reinforcing Partnership

Dr. Klein:
I'm going to be here with you as we go through this.

(Simple. Direct. Anchoring.)

The Teaching Point

Patients do not expect certainty, but they do need direction. Without direction, honesty feels like abandonment. Without honesty, hope feels false. The provider's role is to bridge the two.

What the Patient Leaves With

Not denial, not despair, but something more sustainable:

- An understanding of reality
- A sense that action is still possible
- The knowledge that they are not facing this alone

And in that balance, hope becomes something real—not imagined, not promised, but *held*.

Invite Questions, Gently

Instead of asking, *"Do you have any questions?"*, which often leads to silence, try: "What questions are coming to mind right now?" or "What would you like me to go over again?" This acknowledges that questions are expected, even if the patient cannot yet fully form them. The diagnosis has been delivered. The patient has reacted. Information has been paced, and a direction has been established.

Now comes a subtle but decisive moment. Many providers, almost automatically, ask: "Do you have any questions?" And just as often, the patient responds: "No… I don't think so." Not because they understand everything. But because they are overwhelmed, unsure where to begin, or hesitant to appear uninformed. The way the question is asked determines whether the patient engages—or withdraws.

The Scenario

Dr. Lawson (calm, present):
We've talked about what the diagnosis is, and the next step with the CT scan.

(A brief pause. The patient is quiet, absorbing.)

The Common Approach (and Its Failure)

Dr. Lawson (quickly):
Do you have any questions?

Patient (almost reflexively):
No… I think I'm okay.

(But their expression suggests otherwise. Their silence is not clarity—it is overload.)

Resetting the Approach: The Gentle Invitation

(Dr. Lawson recognizes the moment. He slows down and reframes).

Dr. Lawson (softer, more intentional):
What questions are coming to mind right now?

(The wording assumes there are questions. It removes pressure to "have the right one.")

Patient (after a pause):
I guess… I don't really understand how serious this is.

Why This Works

The patient did not initially ask this question. Not because it wasn't important—but because they needed permission to enter the conversation.

A Second Approach

(Later in the same encounter)

Dr. Lawson:
We've covered a lot in a short time. *(Acknowledging cognitive overload.)*
What would you like me to go over again?

Patient:
Can you explain the scan part again? I didn't really follow that.

What Changed

The provider did not test the patient. He supported them. He made it acceptable to:

- Not understand everything
- Need repetition
- Ask imperfect or incomplete questions

The Emotional Layer

Patients often hesitate to ask questions because they are:

- Afraid of the answer
- Embarrassed to admit confusion
- Trying to appear composed

A gentle invitation lowers all three barriers.

A More Fragile Moment

Patient (quietly):
I don't even know what to ask.

Dr. Lawson (steady):
That's completely okay.

(Pause.)

We can take this one step at a time. I can also walk you through the next part again, if that helps.

The Teaching Point

Inviting questions is not a formality. It is a continuation of care. The goal is not to check a box. It is to open a door.

What the Patient Experiences

Instead of feeling tested, they feel guided. Instead of feeling inadequate, they feel included. And instead of leaving silently confused, they leave with clarity that they helped shape.

The Principle to Remember

Patients rarely ask better questions because they are told to. They ask better questions when they feel safe enough to begin.

The Final Responsibility: Do Not Disappear

One of the most damaging experiences for patients is receiving bad news and then feeling left alone. Before ending the encounter, reinforce continuity with simple, grounding statements such as "I will be here to guide you through this" or "We will take this one step at a time." Even when multiple specialists become involved, the patient should feel that someone remains anchored to them.

The diagnosis has been delivered.
The patient has reacted.
Information has been paced.
Questions have begun.

Now comes the final—and often overlooked—moment: the ending. This is where the patient silently asks, *What happens to me when you walk out of this room?*

The Scenario

Dr. Morgan (calm, present):
We've talked about the diagnosis and the next steps with imaging and oncology.

(The patient sits quietly, absorbing. There is fatigue now, not just shock.)

The Risk of Disappearing

Many encounters end here—with a summary, a nod, and an exit. But without reinforcement, the patient leaves with something dangerous: a sense of being *handed off*, rather than *held within a process.*

The Provider Anchors the Relationship

Dr. Morgan (slowing down, deliberate):
I want you to know something important.

(This signals that what follows matters.)

I will be here to guide you through this.

(He does not rush past the statement.)

Patient (looking up):
...You will?

Making Continuity Explicit

Dr. Morgan:
Yes. You'll be meeting with specialists, and we'll bring in a team to take care of you.

(Pause.)

But I'm not stepping away. I'll stay involved, and we'll move through this together.

The Patient Tests the Meaning

Patient:
So... I'm not just being sent somewhere else?

Dr. Morgan (steady):
No.

(Simple. Clear.)

You're being supported by more people—but you're not losing me in the process.

Reinforcing Structure and Direction

Dr. Morgan:
We're going to take this one step at a time.

(A familiar phrase, now reinforced with context.)

After your scan, we'll sit down again and go through everything together before making any decisions.

Why This Matters

The introduction of specialists can feel, to a patient, like fragmentation:

- New faces
- New language
- New uncertainty

Without an anchor, the experience becomes disorienting.

The Anchor Is Not Control—It Is Presence

The provider does not need to manage every detail, but they must remain visible, accessible, and connected.

A More Vulnerable Response

Patient (quietly):
I was afraid I'd just be… on my own with all of this.

Dr. Morgan (gently):
You won't be.

(Pause.)

We're going to walk through this together.

The Closing Moment

(Dr. Morgan stands, but does not rush.)

Dr. Morgan:
My office will help coordinate the next appointments. And I'll see you again after your scan—we'll go over everything in detail.

(A final moment of eye contact.)

What the Patient Leaves With

Not just a diagnosis, not just a plan, but a *sense of continuity.*

The Teaching Point

Bad news does not end when the information is delivered. It extends into what the patient believes happens next. If the provider disappears, even subtly, the patient feels abandoned within the truth. If the provider remains present—clearly and intentionally—the patient feels guided, even in uncertainty.

What the Patient Remembers

They may not recall the exact staging. They may not remember every treatment option discussed. But they will remember:

- Whether you looked at them when you spoke
- Whether your words were clear or confusing
- Whether you allowed them space to react
- Whether they felt supported—or alone

Delivering bad news is not about softening reality. It is about delivering reality in a way the patient can actually receive. Clarity gives them understanding. Pacing gives them capacity. Emotional awareness gives them stability. And in that moment, stability is everything. This final moment is not about what the provider says next. It is about what remains with the patient after the encounter is over. Not the data. Not the terminology. But the *impression of the experience.*

The Scenario

The conversation has ended. The provider has delivered the diagnosis, paced the information, invited questions, and reinforced continuity.

Now the patient sits quietly for a moment before leaving.

Patient (standing slowly):
Thank you… for explaining everything.

Dr. Chen (gentle, steady):
Of course.

(He maintains eye contact. No glance at the computer. No reaching for the door yet.)

What the Patient Is Processing

At this point, the patient does *not* replay:

- The exact staging terminology
- The detailed treatment pathways
- The sequence of diagnostic steps

Instead, something simpler—and more powerful—forms:

The Internal Experience (Unspoken)

He looked at me when he spoke. He didn't rush me. He told me the truth clearly. He didn't leave me alone with it.

A Subtle Reinforcement

Dr. Chen:
We'll take this one step at a time.

(A familiar phrase now carries emotional weight because it has been consistently supported throughout the interaction.)

Patient (nods):
Okay.

The Exit

(The patient leaves the room. The clinical details begin to blur almost immediately.)

But what remains is not confusion. It is not isolation. It is a *felt sense*:

- I was seen
- I was told the truth
- I was supported

Why This Matters

Memory under stress does not function normally. Details fragment. Information fades. But emotional impressions persist with clarity.

The Contrast

If the same diagnosis had been delivered with:

- Minimal eye contact
- Rushed explanation
- No space for reaction
- A quick exit

The patient might leave with:

- The same information
- But a completely different experience

One that feels cold, confusing, and isolating.

The Integration of the Principles

What the patient remembers is shaped by three forces:

- **Clarity:** They understood what was said, even if not every detail
- **Pacing:** They were not overwhelmed beyond their ability to process
- **Emotional Awareness:** They felt recognized and not alone

The Final Teaching Point

Delivering bad news is not about protecting the patient from reality. It is about making reality *receivable*. Because if reality is delivered without structure or awareness, it becomes noise, fear, and confusion. But if it is delivered with intention, it becomes something the patient can begin to carry.

The Principle to Carry Forward

Long after the specifics are forgotten, the patient remembers one essential truth: How did you make them feel in the moment their world changed? And in that moment, -stability is everything.

Chapter 10

When the Diagnosis Is Uncertain

Communicating Without Eroding Confidence

Uncertainty is one of the most uncomfortable realities in medicine. Not only for patients, but for providers as well. There is a natural impulse to resolve it quickly, to offer a definitive answer, to restore a sense of control.

But uncertainty handled poorly does something subtle and damaging. It erodes confidence. Not because the provider lacks answers, but because the *way uncertainty is communicated* can feel like a lack of direction, a lack of competence, or even a lack of concern. Handled correctly, however, uncertainty can do the opposite. It can build trust.

The Scenario

A patient has ongoing neurological symptoms. MRI and initial labs are inconclusive.

Dr. Stein (seated, composed, direct eye contact):
I want to walk you through where things stand right now.

(This signals structure, not confusion.)

Establishing Ground Before Uncertainty

Dr. Stein:
The MRI did not show anything like a tumor or stroke, which is reassuring.

(He begins with what is known. The patient exhales slightly.)

Naming the Uncertainty Clearly

Dr. Stein:
At the same time, we don't yet have a single clear explanation for your symptoms.

Patient (leans forward):
So… you're not sure what this is?

The Critical Moment

This is where confidence can be lost—or strengthened.

The Provider Protects Confidence

Dr. Stein (steady, calm):
We don't have the final answer yet.

(pause)

But we are not without direction.

Providing Structure Instead of Ambiguity

Dr. Stein:
There are a few specific conditions we're considering based on your symptoms. The next step is to run more focused tests to narrow that down.

Patient:
Okay… so this isn't just… guessing?

Reassurance Through Process, Not False Certainty

Dr. Stein:
No. This is a step-by-step process.

(He leans slightly forward.)

We've ruled out the most urgent causes. Now we're working through the more subtle ones in a systematic way.

The Patient Begins to Stabilize

Patient (nods slowly):
That makes sense…

Addressing the Emotional Undercurrent

Patient:
It's just hard not knowing.

Dr. Stein (acknowledging, not dismissing):
I understand that.

(pause)

Not having an answer yet can feel unsettling. My role is to make sure we keep moving forward until we do.

Reinforcing Ongoing Engagement

Dr. Stein:
And I'll be following this closely with you. You're not navigating this on your own.

A Subtle Shift Occurs

The uncertainty has not changed. But the *experience* of it has.

What Would Have Eroded Confidence

Compare this to a different approach: "I'm not really sure what's going on. We'll just have to see." That statement may be honest—but it feels:

- Directionless
- Passive
- Detached

What Built Confidence Instead

Dr. Stein communicated four things clearly:

- What is known
- What is not yet known
- What is being done next
- That he remains engaged

The Teaching Point

Uncertainty does not undermine confidence. Unstructured uncertainty does. When the provider:

- Names it clearly
- Frames it logically

- Provides next steps
- Remains present

The patient does not feel lost. They feel guided.

The Principle to Remember

You do not need to have the final answer to inspire confidence. You need to show that:

- There is a path.
- You are on it.
- And the patient is not walking it alone.

The Core Principle

Patients do not expect you to know everything. They expect you to know how to think, how to proceed, and how to stay engaged. Uncertainty becomes dangerous only when it feels unmanaged.

The Scenario

A patient presents with persistent abdominal pain. Initial labs and imaging are inconclusive.

Dr. Mehta (sitting, composed)**:**
I want to go over what we know so far, and what we don't yet know.

(This immediately creates structure.)

Step One: Establish What Is Known

Dr. Mehta:
Your blood work looks normal, and the CT scan did not show anything urgent or immediately dangerous.

(Clear. Grounding. This reduces fear before introducing uncertainty.)

Step Two: Name the Uncertainty Clearly

Dr. Mehta:
At the same time, we don't yet have a clear explanation for the pain you've been experiencing.

(No evasion. No false certainty.)

Patient (slightly tense)**:**
So… you don't know what's causing it?

Step Three: Protect Confidence While Acknowledging Limits

Dr. Mehta (steady):
We don't have the full answer yet.

(Pause.)

But we do have a clear plan for how to find it.

Why This Matters

The phrase *"I don't know"* alone can feel like a dead end. But *"We don't know yet—and here is what we're doing next"* creates direction.

Step Four: Provide a Structured Plan

Dr. Mehta:
The next step is to look more closely at how your digestive system is functioning. I'd like to order an endoscopy and also adjust a few things to see how your symptoms respond.

(Specific. Forward moving.)

The Patient Regains Stability

Patient:
Okay… so there's still a path to figure this out.

Dr. Mehta:
Exactly.

Step Five: Set Expectations Without Alarm

Dr. Mehta:
Sometimes these things take a few steps to fully understand. What's important is that we're ruling out serious causes and moving in a logical direction.

What Was Avoided

The provider did not say:

- "Everything looks fine" (which dismisses the patient's experience)
- "It's probably nothing" (which can feel minimizing)
- "I'm not sure" without follow-through (which feels uncertain and incomplete)

A More Complex Scenario — When Serious Conditions Are Still Possible

Dr. Mehta:

There are a few possibilities we're considering. Some are minor, and some are more serious.

(Balanced framing.)

We don't have evidence of anything dangerous right now, but we're continuing to evaluate carefully to be sure.

Why This Works

- It does not falsely reassure
- It does not alarm prematurely
- It communicates vigilance and responsibility

The Emotional Layer

Uncertainty often triggers anxiety not because of the unknown itself, but because of what the patient imagines filling that unknown. Your role is not to eliminate uncertainty. It is to contain it.

Containing Uncertainty in One Sentence

"We don't have the full answer yet, but we are actively working through it, and I will guide you step by step."

The Teaching Point

Confidence is not built by having all the answers. It is built by demonstrating:

- Clear thinking
- Honest communication
- A structured plan
- Continued presence

What the Patient Leaves With

Not certainty. But something just as important:

- A sense that nothing critical is being missed
- A clear understanding of what comes next
- Confidence that the provider is engaged and in control of the process

The Principle to Remember

Uncertainty is unavoidable. But unmanaged uncertainty feels like abandonment. When you name it, structure it, and stay present within it, uncertainty becomes not a weakness, but a space the provider actively holds and shapes.

A Final Integrated Dialogue

This is the moment where everything comes together. Not a technique. Not a script. But a way of *holding uncertainty* so that the patient does not feel lost inside it.

The Scenario

A patient has ongoing symptoms. Multiple tests have been done. Nothing definitive has emerged.

Dr. Ellison (calm, seated, grounded)**:**
I want to talk through where we are right now.

Naming the Reality Clearly

Dr. Ellison:
We've done several important tests, and so far, we have not found a single clear diagnosis that explains everything you're experiencing.

(The patient shifts slightly. There is tension—but also attention.)

Avoiding the Pitfall of Unmanaged Uncertainty

Patient:
So… you don't know what this is?

The Provider Holds Structure

Dr. Ellison (steady):
We don't have the final answer yet.

(Pause.)

But we do understand a lot more than we did before.

Creating Orientation

Dr. Ellison:
We've ruled out the most serious and urgent conditions. That's important.

(The patient exhales slightly.)

What we're doing now is narrowing down the remaining possibilities in a careful, step-by-step way.

Turning Uncertainty Into Process

Patient:
So there's still a plan?

Dr. Ellison:
Yes. There is a clear plan.

(Leaning slightly forward.)

The next step is to focus on how your symptoms are evolving and run a more targeted set of tests based on that.

Addressing the Emotional Weight

Patient (quietly)**:**
It's just hard not knowing.

Dr. Ellison (acknowledging)**:**
I understand.

(Pause.)

Not having a name for something yet can feel unsettling.

Staying Present Within the Uncertainty

Dr. Ellison:
But you're not in this alone.

(Simple. Direct.)

I'm going to stay with you through this process, and we're going to keep moving forward until we have answers.

The Shift

The uncertainty has not disappeared. But it has changed form. It is no longer:

- A void
- A gap
- A source of quiet panic

It is now:

- A process
- A direction
- A shared effort

What the Patient Now Holds

Not certainty, but something steadier:

- *Nothing critical has been missed*
- *There is a plan in motion*
- *My provider is engaged and not stepping away*

The Final Teaching Point

Uncertainty is not the enemy. What patients fear is being left *inside* it without guidance. When you:

- Name it clearly
- Structure it thoughtfully
- Stay present within it

You transform uncertainty from something that erodes trust into something that builds it.

The Principle

Uncertainty is unavoidable. But when it is carried with clarity, structure, and presence, it becomes not a weakness but a visible expression of disciplined, reliable care.

Chapter 11

Managing Patient Anxiety and Fear

Practical Approaches to Emotional Regulation

Anxiety in the clinical setting is not an obstacle to care. It is a signal. It tells you that the patient's sense of safety has been disrupted. That their mind is moving faster than their ability to process. That fear is beginning to organize their thinking.

When anxiety rises, information alone is not enough. In fact, more information—delivered too quickly—can intensify it. The provider's role in these moments is not to eliminate fear. It is to regulate the environment, the pace, and the interaction so that the patient can regain enough stability to think, listen, and engage. Anxiety has already entered the room. It is not subtle. It is visible in the patient's voice, posture, and pace. The provider's role is not to argue with it. It is to regulate what surrounds it.

The Scenario

Patient (fast, restless, voice elevated):
I don't understand why this is happening. The pain keeps coming back, and nobody's given me a clear answer. What if something's being missed? What if this is serious?

Step One: Regulate the Pace

Dr. Malik (slower, grounded tone):
Let's slow this down for a moment.

(He does not match the patient's speed. He deliberately reduces it.)

Step Two: Acknowledge the Emotional State

Dr. Malik:
I can see how much this has been weighing on you.

Patient (still tense, but slightly quieter):
It has… I can't stop thinking about it.

Step Three: Contain the Experience

Dr. Malik:
Right now, your mind is trying to make sense of something that doesn't yet have a clear answer.

(This normalizes the reaction without dismissing it.)

Step Four: Create Immediate Structure

Dr. Malik (gently redirecting):
Let's focus on where we are right now.

(Pause.)

You're here. We've done initial tests. And we're working through this step by step.

The Shift Begins

The patient's breathing slows slightly.
Not because the fear is gone—but because it now has boundaries.

Step Five: Limit Information to What Can Be Held

Patient:
But what if it's something really serious?

Dr. Malik (measured)**:**
That's a possibility your mind is going to go to.

(Pause.)

Right now, based on what we've seen, there's no indication of anything dangerous. But we are continuing to evaluate carefully.

Step Six: Anchor to the Next Action

Dr. Malik:
The next step is the imaging study we scheduled. That will give us more clarity.

(Pause.)

Let's focus on that step first.

Step Seven: Use Presence as Regulation

(Dr. Malik remains still. No typing. No distraction.)

Dr. Malik:
You're not dealing with this alone.

A More Heightened Moment

Patient (voice shaking):
I just feel like I'm losing control over this.

Dr. Malik (calm, grounded):
That feeling makes sense.

(Pause.)

So, let's bring it back to what we can control right now.

(Slight lean forward.)

We're evaluating this carefully. We have a plan. And we're moving forward.

What Just Happened

The provider did not:

- Flood the patient with more data
- Dismiss the concern
- Attempt to eliminate fear

Instead, he:

- Slowed the pace
- Acknowledged the emotion
- Created structure
- Anchored the present
- Maintained presence

The Internal Shift in the Patient

From:

- Racing thoughts
- Catastrophic projection
- Loss of control

To:

- Focused attention
- Contained concern
- Shared direction

The Teaching Point

Anxiety is not resolved through explanation alone. It is regulated through environment, pacing, and presence.

The Principle to Remember

You are not trying to remove fear. You are creating conditions in which fear does not overwhelm the patient's ability to think. When the patient regains even a small degree of stability, they can begin to listen, understand, and engage again. And that is where care becomes possible.

The First Principle: Slow the Room Before You Speak

An anxious patient often speaks quickly, breathes shallowly, and jumps between concerns. If the provider matches that pace, anxiety escalates. If the provider *slows down*, the room begins to recalibrate.

Regulating the Room Through Pace — A Dialogue Contrast That Sticks

This is one of the most important—and most overlooked—skills in patient interaction. Not what you say, but how fast you say it.

Scenario: Same Patient, Two Different Providers

A patient arrives visibly anxious.

Version One: Matching the Patient's Pace (Escalation)

Patient (rapid, tense):
I just don't understand what's going on—this keeps happening, and what if it's something serious? What if something's being missed?

Dr. Lee (quick, reactive):
Okay, okay—so the labs were normal, the imaging didn't show anything, we can run more tests if needed, but nothing stands out right now—

Patient (interrupting, more anxious)**:**
But then why is this happening? That doesn't make sense!

Dr. Lee (speaking faster):
Well, sometimes these things don't show up right away, but we can refer you, maybe repeat imaging, check more labs—

What Just Happened

- The provider matched the patient's speed
- The conversation became compressed and fragmented
- Anxiety fed on itself

The patient leaves with more information—but less stability.

Version Two: Slowing the Pace (Regulation)

Patient (rapid, tense):
I just don't understand what's going on—this keeps happening, and what if it's something serious? What if something's being missed?

Dr. Lee (slower, grounded):
Let's slow this down for a moment.

(Pause. The first interruption of momentum.)

Dr. Lee (calm, measured):
I can see how concerning this has been for you.

Patient (breathing begins to settle slightly):
Yeah... it really has.

Dr. Lee:
Let's take this one step at a time.

(Another pause. The room continues to decelerate.)

Now the Information Can Land

Dr. Lee:
The tests we've done so far have not shown anything dangerous.

(Pause.)

And we're continuing to evaluate this carefully.

Patient (quieter now):
Okay...

What Changed

Nothing about the medical facts changed. Only the pace.

The Invisible Mechanism

When the provider slows:

- The patient's breathing begins to match
- The cognitive load decreases
- Emotional intensity lowers just enough for thinking to return

This is not psychological theory in the abstract. It is observable in real time.

The Teaching Point

If you match anxiety, you amplify it. If you regulate pace, you contain it.

The Principle to Remember

The room will always take on the rhythm of the provider. When you slow down deliberately—your voice, your pauses, your movement—you are not just communicating differently. You are changing the patient's physiological state. And in that shift, the patient regains enough steadiness to hear you, think with you, and move forward.

The Second Principle: Name the Anxiety Without Amplifying It

Avoid dismissing anxiety ("You're fine") or fueling it ("This could be anything"). Instead, acknowledge what is present.

A Dialogue That Demonstrates the Shift

Anxiety does not need to be corrected. It needs to be recognized accurately. If dismissed, the patient feels minimized. If amplified, the patient feels overwhelmed. The provider's task is to land in the narrow space between the two.

Scenario

The patient is visibly tense. Their thoughts are moving quickly, and their concern is escalating.

Patient (tight, uneasy):
I just can't stop thinking about this. What if something is seriously wrong? I mean, what if we're missing something important?

What Not to Do (Dismissal)

Dr. Rao (too quickly):
You're fine. There's nothing to worry about.

Patient (pulls back slightly):
...Okay.

(But internally, nothing has changed. The anxiety is now unspoken—but still present.)

What Not to Do (Amplification)

Dr. Rao (overly serious tone):
Well, there are a lot of possibilities. It could be a number of things.

Patient (eyes widen):
Like what?

(Anxiety increases. The mind fills the gaps with worst-case scenarios.)

The Correct Approach: Naming What Is Present

Dr. Rao (calm, grounded):
I can hear how much this has been worrying you.

(A pause. The patient exhales slightly.)

Patient:
Yeah… it's been on my mind constantly.

What Just Happened

Nothing about the diagnosis changed. No new information was introduced. But something shifted:

- The patient felt *seen*
- The internal tension decreased slightly
- The conversation became more grounded

Going One Step Further

Dr. Rao:
When something doesn't have a clear answer yet, it's natural for your mind to go to those places.

(This normalizes without reinforcing fear.)

Patient (nods):
Exactly… that's what's happening.

Why This Works

The provider did not:

- Deny the anxiety
- Feed the anxiety
- Try to immediately solve it

Instead, he accurately reflected it.

The Subtle Skill

Notice the language:

- "I can hear..." (not "You are...")
- "This has been worrying you." (not "You should be worried.")

It stays anchored in observation, not interpretation.

The Teaching Point

Anxiety decreases the moment it feels recognized. Not fixed. Not argued with. Recognized.

The Principle to Remember

When you name anxiety correctly, you are telling the patient something powerful without saying it directly: "I see what's happening inside you, and you are not alone in it." And in that moment, the intensity of the fear begins—quietly—to loosen.

The Third Principle: Create Structure to Contain Fear

Anxiety thrives in ambiguity. Structure reduces it.

A Dialogue That Builds Stability

Fear expands in open space. When there is no structure, the patient fills the gaps with imagination—often worst-case scenarios. Structure does not eliminate uncertainty. It gives the mind something to hold on to.

Scenario

The patient remains anxious. Their thoughts are scattered, moving between possibilities and fears.

Patient (uneasy, searching):
I just don't know what to think anymore... every time I feel something, I assume the worst.

Without Structure (Ambiguity Persists)

Dr. Rao (vague):
We're still looking into things.

Patient (frustrated, unsettled):
But what does that mean?

(Ambiguity increases anxiety. There is no anchor.)

Introducing Structure

Dr. Rao (calm, deliberate):
Let me walk you through what we know so far, and what we're doing next.

(A pause. The tone shifts from uncertainty to guidance.)

Step One: What Is Known

Dr. Rao:
So far, your tests have not shown anything dangerous or urgent.

(The patient's posture softens slightly.)

Step Two: What Is Not Yet Known

Dr. Rao:
At the same time, we don't yet have a single clear explanation for your symptoms.

(This is honest—but now placed within structure, not left open-ended.)

Step Three: What Comes Next

Dr. Rao:
The next step is to run a more focused test that looks specifically at how your system is functioning.

(Pause.)

We'll use that information to guide what we do after that.

The Patient Reorients

Patient (leans forward slightly):
Okay… so there's a plan.

Dr. Rao:
Yes. We're moving through this step by step.

What Just Happened

The uncertainty did not disappear. But it was contained. The patient moved from "Anything could be wrong" to "There is a process unfolding."

Why Structure Works

Structure does three things simultaneously:

1. Reduces ambiguity
2. Creates predictability
3. Restores a sense of direction

The Subtle Shift in the Patient

Instead of scanning for danger, the patient begins to follow the process.

The Teaching Point

When anxiety is high, the patient is not asking for more information. They are asking for organization.

The Principle to Remember

You do not calm fear by saying less. You calm fear by organizing what is happening. When you say: "Here is what we know. Here is what we don't yet know. Here is what we are doing next," you replace chaos with structure. And in that structure, the patient finds just enough stability to move forward.

The Fourth Principle: Separate Possibility from Probability

Anxious patients often fixate on worst-case scenarios. The provider must gently recalibrate this without dismissing concern.

A Dialogue That Recalibrates Fear

Anxious patients do not think in probabilities. They think in possibilities. And when fear is present, the mind gravitates toward the most serious possibility—not the most likely one. The provider's role is not to dismiss that fear, but to gently bring it back into proportion.

Scenario

Patient (concerned, searching):
What if this is something really serious?

The Wrong Direction: Dismissal

Dr. Rao (too quickly):
It's nothing serious.

(The patient may nod—but internally, doubt grows. The concern has been dismissed, not addressed.)

The Wrong Direction: Amplification

Dr. Rao (overly cautious tone):
Well, we can't rule anything out.

(The patient's fear expands. The worst-case scenario now feels equally likely.)

The Correct Approach: Calibrating Possibility vs. Probability

Dr. Rao (measured, steady): That's an understandable concern.

(Pause. The fear is acknowledged, not dismissed.)

Dr. Rao (continues):
Right now, based on what we've seen, the likelihood of something serious is low.

(Another pause. This is the recalibration.)

Dr. Rao:
But we're still evaluating carefully to be sure.

What Just Happened

The provider did three things simultaneously:

- Validated the fear without reinforcing it
- Introduced perspective grounded in evidence
- Maintained vigilance to preserve trust

The Patient's Internal Shift

From:

- "This could be something terrible."

To:

- "That's possible, but not likely—and it's being checked."

Extending the Dialogue

Patient (quieter):
So you don't think it's something dangerous?

Dr. Rao:
Based on what we have right now, there's nothing pointing in that direction.

(Pause.)

And we're continuing to look carefully so we don't miss anything.

Why This Works

The patient is not being told what to feel. They are being given a framework to think.

The Teaching Point

Fear distorts probability. It elevates rare outcomes into perceived inevitabilities. Your role is to gently restore proportion—without invalidating the concern.

The Principle to Remember

You are not eliminating the possibility. You are clarifying the likelihood. And when you do that with:

- Calm acknowledgment
- Clear perspective
- Ongoing vigilance

You replace catastrophic thinking with grounded understanding. And that shift is what allows the patient to regain a sense of balance.

The Fifth Principle: Anchor the Patient in the Next Step

Anxiety often projects into an uncertain future. Grounding happens in the immediate next action.

A Dialogue That Grounds the Future

Anxiety pulls the patient forward—into imagined outcomes, worst-case scenarios, and unanswered questions. The mind runs ahead faster than reality can keep up. The provider's role is to gently bring the patient back—not to the entire future, but to the very next step.

Scenario

Patient (tense, overwhelmed):
I just keep thinking… what if this gets worse? What if it turns into something serious? What happens then?

The Risk: Following the Patient into the Future

Dr. Rao (too broad):
Well, if it's serious, we might need more tests, maybe treatment, possibly specialists…

(The patient's anxiety increases. The future expands into multiple unknowns.)

The Correct Approach: Anchoring the Present

Dr. Rao (steady, focused):
The next step is the ultrasound we scheduled.

(Pause. The scope narrows immediately.)

Dr. Rao (continues)**:**
"That will give us more specific information about what's going on."

(Another pause. Let the patient absorb something concrete.)

Dr. Rao (gently redirecting):
Let's focus on that step first.

What Just Happened

The provider did not engage the patient's imagined future. He re-centered the conversation on a single, actionable point.

The Patient's Shift

Patient (breathing steadier):
Okay… so that's the next thing.

Dr. Rao:
Exactly.

Why This Works

Anxiety thrives in:

- Multiple unknowns
- Distant possibilities
- Lack of control

It decreases when the patient can see:

- A clear next action
- A defined timeline
- A sense of movement

Extending the Grounding

Patient:
And after that?

Dr. Rao (still structured):
Once we have the results, we'll sit down and go through them together and decide the next step.

(Still not jumping ahead unnecessarily. Still one step at a time.)

The Teaching Point

You do not calm anxiety by answering every future question. You calm it by limiting the frame.

The Principle to Remember

When the patient is overwhelmed by what *might* happen, bring them back to what *is happening next.* Not the entire path. Not every possibility. Just the next step. And in that step, the patient regains something essential: a sense of direction.

The Sixth Principle: Use the Body to Calm the Mind

Emotional regulation is not only cognitive. It is physiological. Small, subtle cues matter:

- Slower speech
- Pauses
- Steady tone
- Sitting instead of standing

These signals tell the patient's nervous system: *This is contained. This is manageable.*

A Dialogue That Regulates Physiology, Not Just Thought

Anxiety is not only happening in the patient's mind. It is happening in their body: faster breathing, tension in the muscles, a voice that tightens and accelerates. If you speak only to the mind, you miss half the problem. If you regulate the body, the mind begins to follow.

Scenario: Heightened Anxiety

Patient (visibly panicked, speaking quickly):
I can't stop thinking about this. I haven't been sleeping. My mind just keeps going—I feel like I'm losing control over it."

What Not to Do: Stay Cognitive Only

Dr. Rao (too informational):
Well, your tests are normal, and statistically this isn't likely to be serious.

(The patient nods, but their body remains tense. The anxiety is unchanged.)

The Correct Approach: Regulate First, Then Inform

(Dr. Rao sits fully, shoulders relaxed. He slows his breathing before speaking.)

Dr. Rao (gentle, slower cadence)
That sounds exhausting.

(Pause. Not brief—intentional.)

What This Pause Does.

The patient's system begins to mirror the provider's pace. Not consciously—but physiologically.

Dr. Rao (even slower now):
Right now… let's just focus on this moment.

(Another pause. The room becomes quieter.)

You're here.

(Pause.)

We're talking through it.

(Pause.)

And we have a plan in place.

The Patient's Shift

Patient (breathing begins to slow):
…Okay.

What Just Happened

The provider did not:

- Challenge the thoughts directly
- Provide more data
- Attempt to "fix" the anxiety

Instead, he changed:

- His tone
- His pace
- His posture
- His pauses

And the patient's body responded.

The Subtle Tools of Regulation

These are not techniques to memorize. They are signals the patient's nervous system reads instantly:

- Sitting down instead of standing
- Leaning slightly forward, not back
- Speaking slower than feels natural
- Allowing silence without rushing to fill it

Extending the Moment

Patient (quieter now):
I just… feel overwhelmed.

Dr. Rao (steady, grounded):
That makes sense.

(Pause.)

We're going to take this one step at a time.

Why This Works

The body cannot sustain high anxiety in the presence of consistent, calm signals. Over time—even seconds—it begins to downshift.

The Teaching Point

You are not only communicating with words. You are communicating with rhythm, tone, and presence.

The Principle to Remember

When the patient's body is in distress, you must meet it there: slow your voice, slow your movements, allow space. When the body begins to settle, the mind finally becomes able to listen, process, and engage again.

The Seventh Principle: Do Not Rush Reassurance

Premature reassurance often backfires. Saying "Everything will be fine" may feel comforting in the moment, but if uncertainty remains, it weakens trust. Instead, offer grounded reassurance.

A Dialogue That Builds Trust Instead of False Comfort

Reassurance is one of the most natural instincts in medicine. When a patient is anxious, the impulse is to relieve that discomfort quickly. But reassurance given too early—or without foundation—does something subtle. It may calm the moment, but it undermines trust over time. Patients are not only listening for comfort. They are listening for *credibility*.

Scenario

Patient (worried, searching):
Do you think I'm going to be okay?

The Common Mistake: Premature Reassurance

Dr. Rao (quickly):
You'll be fine. Don't worry.

The patient nods, but inside something tightens. The reassurance feels too fast, too certain. A quiet doubt surfaces:
How does he know that? What if he's wrong?

The Shift: Grounded Reassurance

Dr. Rao (measured, steady):
We're taking this seriously, and we're working through it carefully.

(Pause. The reassurance is anchored in action, not prediction.)

Why This Works

The provider does not promise an outcome. He communicates:

- Attention
- Responsibility
- Ongoing effort

Extending the Dialogue

Patient:
So… you don't know yet?

Dr. Rao:
We don't have all the answers yet.

(Pause.)

But we're being thorough, and we're moving in a clear direction.

The Emotional Impact

Instead of feeling falsely reassured, the patient feels secure in the process.

A More Fragile Moment

Patient (quietly):
I'm just scared this could turn into something serious.

Dr. Rao (calm, grounded):
I understand that.

(Pause.)

And that's exactly why we're approaching this carefully and not overlooking anything.

What Was Avoided

The provider did not:

- Dismiss the fear
- Offer certainty he cannot guarantee
- Minimize the situation

The Teaching Point

Reassurance should not be about predicting the future. It should be about demonstrating reliability in the present.

The Principle to Remember

False reassurance says: "Everything will be fine." Grounded reassurance says: "You are being carefully and thoughtfully cared for." And when patients believe that, they do not need certainty to feel stable.

The Eighth Principle: Reinforce Ongoing Presence

Anxiety decreases when the patient feels they are not alone in managing it.

A Dialogue That Prevents Isolation

Anxiety does not come only from symptoms. It comes from the feeling of being left alone with them. Even when a plan exists, even when tests are scheduled, a patient can still feel unanchored if they sense that no one is *actively with them* in the process. Presence, when made explicit, reduces that isolation.

Scenario

The visit is nearing its end. The plan has been discussed. The patient is quieter now—but still uneasy.

Patient (hesitant):
So... I just wait for the test?

The Risk: Passive Framing

Dr. Rao (neutral):
Yes, we'll see what it shows.

(Technically correct—but emotionally incomplete. The patient is left alone in the waiting.)

The Correct Approach: Reinforcing Presence

Dr. Rao (steady, intentional):
I'll be following this closely with you.

(Pause. This is not a routine statement—it is a commitment.)

Dr. Rao (continues):
If anything changes, or if your concerns increase, we'll address it together.

The Patient's Shift

Patient (relaxes slightly):
Okay… that helps.

What Just Happened

Nothing about the timeline changed. Nothing about the uncertainty changed. But something essential did:

- The patient is no longer waiting alone.
- They are being followed.

Extending the Presence

Dr. Rao:
After your test, we'll go over the results together and decide the next step.

(This reinforces continuity—not just availability.)

A More Vulnerable Moment

Patient (quietly):
I just don't want this to get worse and not know what to do.

Dr. Rao (calm, direct):
You won't be handling that on your own.

(Pause.)

If anything changes, you reach out—and we'll respond together.

Why This Works

Anxiety decreases when:

- The patient knows who is responsible
- The patient knows they are being monitored
- The patient feels included in a shared process

The Teaching Point

Presence must be stated, not assumed. Patients cannot feel what is not made visible.

The Principle to Remember

You are not only managing a condition. You are managing the patient's experience of going through it. When you say: "I will be following this with you," you replace uncertainty with connection. And in that connection, the patient finds something deeply stabilizing: They are not alone in what comes next.

What the Patient Experiences

When done correctly, the patient does not leave without fear, but they leave with something more important:

- Their fear is **contained**, not spiraling
- Their thinking is **organized**, not scattered
- Their care feels **guided**, not uncertain

A Final Integrative Dialogue

This is not a single moment. It is the result of everything that came before—pace, clarity, structure, presence. The goal was never to eliminate fear. It was to change the patient's relationship to it.

The Scenario

The visit is ending. The patient has asked questions, heard the plan, and processed what they can.

Patient (quieter now, reflective):
I'm still worried… but I feel like I understand things better.

Dr. Rao (steady, grounded):
That makes sense.

(Pause.)

There's still uncertainty—but we've put structure around it.

What the Patient Is Actually Experiencing

Not the absence of fear, but a shift in how that fear behaves.

The Patient Names It

Patient:
Before, my mind was just going everywhere… now it feels more… manageable.

Dr. Rao:
That's exactly what we want.

The Three Internal Shifts

Without stating them directly, the patient is now experiencing:

1. Fear is Contained, Not Spiraling

Patient:
I'm not jumping to the worst-case scenario as much.

Dr. Rao:
We've narrowed the focus. That helps keep things grounded.

2. Thinking Is Organized, Not Scattered

Patient:
I know what's happening next… that makes a difference.

Dr. Rao:
One step at a time keeps it clear.

3. Care Feels Guided, Not Uncertain

Patient (after a pause):
I don't feel like I'm just… waiting and hoping.

Dr. Rao:
You're not. We're actively working through this together.

The Closing Moment

(The patient stands, more composed than when they entered.)

Patient:
Thank you… I really needed this explained this way.

Dr. Rao:
Of course.

(Maintains eye contact.)

We'll take the next step together.

What Was Achieved

The diagnosis may still be unclear. The outcome may still be unknown. But the patient leaves with:

- a contained emotional state
- a structured understanding
- a sense of guided care

The Teaching Point

You are not measured only by the answers you provide. You are measured by what the patient is able to carry when they leave.

The Principle to Remember

A patient can leave with uncertainty and still feel stable, but a patient who leaves overwhelmed cannot engage in their own care. When done correctly, you have not removed fear, you have made it manageable, organized, and shared. And that is what allows the patient to move forward.

The Teaching Point

You are not trying to remove anxiety. You are helping the patient regulate within it. Because a regulated patient can:

- Listen
- Understand
- Participate

An overwhelmed patient cannot.

The Principle to Remember

Anxiety accelerates. Your role is to decelerate. When you slow the pace, create structure, and remain present, you do not just deliver care—you make it possible for the patient to receive it.

Chapter 12

The Angry or Distrustful Patient

De-escalation Without Defensiveness

Anger in the clinical setting is rarely about anger alone. It is often the visible edge of something deeper: fear, loss of control, prior negative experiences, or a growing sense that something is not being heard or taken seriously. Distrust, similarly, is not usually born in the moment. It is carried into the room—sometimes from past encounters, sometimes from the system itself.

When a patient presents with anger or distrust, the instinct to defend, correct, or regain control is strong. But defensiveness, even when subtle, escalates the interaction. In that moment, something immediate happens internally for the provider. A tightening. A readiness to explain, to justify, to correct.

That instinct is natural. But it is also the point at which the interaction either escalates—or stabilizes. The provider's task is not to win the exchange. It is to stabilize it.

Understanding What Is Really Present

Anger, in the clinical setting, is rarely about the surface issue alone. It often represents:

- Fear that has not been acknowledged
- A loss of control over one's own body
- Prior experiences of being dismissed or overlooked
- A growing belief that no one is truly listening

Distrust follows a similar path. It is not created in a single sentence. It accumulates—sometimes from previous providers, sometimes from the system itself. So, when a patient says: "No one here knows what they're doing," what may actually be present is: *"I don't feel safe in this process."*

The Critical Mistake: Defensiveness

When the provider responds with:

- justification ("We've been very busy."),

- correction ("That's not accurate."), or
- authority ("You need to trust me."),

the interaction shifts from care to conflict. Even subtle defensiveness communicates something powerful: *"I am protecting myself, not focusing on you."* And the patient feels that immediately.

The Dialogue May Be:

The Escalation Path

Patient (frustrated):
"his is ridiculous. I've been waiting for answers and nobody calls me back.

Provider (defensive tone):
We have a lot of patients. These things take time.

(The patient's frustration sharpens. The conversation becomes oppositional.)

The Stabilizing Path

Patient (frustrated):
This is ridiculous. I've been waiting for answers and nobody calls me back.

Provider (calm, grounded):
I can hear how frustrating that's been.

(Pause. No correction. No defense.)

Patient (still tense, but less sharp)**:**
Of course it's frustrating. I don't know what's going on.

Provider:
You've been left without clear information—and that's not a good place to be.

(Alignment, not opposition.)

What Just Happened

The provider did not agree with everything that was said, but they validated the experience without endorsing the accusation. That distinction is critical.

Stabilization Through Structure

Once the emotional intensity lowers—even slightly—the provider introduces direction.

Provider:
Let's go through where things are right now, and what we're going to do next.

(The conversation shifts from confrontation to orientation.)

Handling Distrust Directly

Distrust often appears as questioning intent.

Patient:
How do I know I actually need this test? Maybe this is just more unnecessary stuff.

The Defensive Response

Provider:
This is standard. You should follow my recommendation.

The Stabilizing Response

Provider (steady, transparent):
That's a fair question.

(Pause.)

"Let me explain exactly why I'm recommending it and what information it gives us."

Transparency replaces authority. Explanation replaces expectation.

The Internal Discipline Required

De-escalation without defensiveness is not passive. It requires active control over:

- Tone
- Pace
- Language
- Emotional reaction

You are not suppressing your response. You are choosing a different one.

The Turning Point

Every interaction like this has a moment where the patient shifts. It may be subtle:

Patient (quieter):
I just want to understand what's going on.

This is the signal. The anger is no longer leading. The patient is ready to engage.

The Teaching Point

You are not responsible for the patient's initial emotion. But you are responsible for what happens next.

The Principle to Remember

When a patient presents with anger or distrust,

- do not defend,
- do not correct immediately, and
- do not try to "win."

Instead,

- acknowledge the experience,
- stay composed,
- introduce structure, and
- maintain clarity,

because the goal is not to prove that you are right. The goal is to create a space where the patient no longer needs to fight to be heard. And when that happens, the interaction transforms—from conflict to care.

The Core Principle

Anger escalates when it meets resistance. It de-escalates when it meets composure, acknowledgment, and structure.

A Dialogue Demonstrating De-escalation Without Defensiveness

The Scenario

A patient arrives visibly frustrated after waiting for test results.

Patient (sharp, confrontational):
I've been waiting for days. No one called me. Do you people even care what's going on with me?

The Common Reaction: Defensiveness

Dr. Carter (tight tone):
"We've been very busy, and these things take time."

(The patient's frustration increases. The interaction becomes adversarial.)

The Correct Approach: Absorb, Don't Reflect

Dr. Carter (calm, steady):
I can hear how frustrating that's been.

(Pause. No justification. No correction.)

Patient (still tense, but slightly less sharp):
Of course it's frustrating. I'm the one sitting here not knowing what's going on.

Step One: Acknowledge Without Arguing

Dr. Carter:
You're right—you've been waiting without clear information, and that's difficult.

(The provider aligns with the patient's experience, not against it.)

Step Two: Do Not Take the Bait

The patient may continue:

Patient:
This is exactly why I don't trust providers. No one follows through.

This is a critical moment.

Step Three: Stay Grounded, Not Defensive

Dr. Carter (even tone):
I understand why it would feel that way, given your experience.

(No attempt to defend the profession. No correction. Just acknowledgment.)

Step Four: Introduce Structure

Dr. Carter:
Let's focus on where things are right now and what we're going to do next.

(The conversation shifts from emotion alone to direction.)

Step Five: Provide Clarity

Dr. Carter:
Your results are in. I have them here, and I'm going to go through them with you now.

(The patient's attention redirects.)

Step Six: Restore Partnership

Patient (less aggressive):
Okay…

Dr. Carter:
We'll go through this together, and I'll make sure you have a clear understanding before you leave.

A Distrust-Focused Scenario: Meeting Skepticism with Transparency

Distrust does not respond to authority. It responds to clarity, reasoning, and openness. When a patient questions your motives, they are not simply asking about the test. They are asking: *"Are you acting in my interest, or not?"* That question cannot be answered with status or credentials. It must be answered with transparency.

The Scenario

Patient (skeptical, guarded):
How do I know I'm not just being sent for more tests I don't even need?

The Reflex That Fails

Provider (firm, authoritative):
You need to trust me.

(This closes the conversation. The patient feels dismissed, and distrust deepens.)

The Correct Response: Open the Reasoning

Dr. Carter (calm, unhurried):
That's a fair question.

(Pause. This matters. It signals respect, not resistance.)

Dr. Carter (transparent):
Let me explain exactly why I'm recommending this test and what information it gives us.

What This Does Immediately

- Validates the patient's right to question
- Removes the power struggle
- Shifts from authority → explanation

Continuing the Dialogue

Dr. Carter:
Based on your symptoms and what we've seen so far, there are a few possibilities we're trying to sort through.

(Clear, structured reasoning.)

This test helps us determine whether this is something structural or functional. Without it, we'd be making decisions with incomplete information.

Patient (less guarded):
So it's not just routine… it actually tells you something specific?

Dr. Carter:
Exactly. It gives us information we don't currently have, and that helps us avoid guessing.

The Shift

The patient is no longer challenging the provider. They are engaging with the reasoning.

A Deeper Layer of Distrust

Sometimes the concern is not just about necessity; it is about intent.

Patient:
I just don't want to be put through things I don't need.

Dr. Carter (direct, steady):
I understand that.

(Pause.)

My goal is the same as yours—to get the right information with the least unnecessary steps.

Why This Works

The provider aligns goals with the patient. Not "my plan" vs. "your concern," but a shared objective.

The Teaching Point

Distrust is not reduced by insisting on trust. It is reduced by making your thinking visible.

The Principle to Remember

When a patient questions you, they are not undermining your authority; they are asking to understand your judgment. When you respond with

- calm acknowledgment,
- clear reasoning,
- transparent intent,

you replace suspicion with understanding. And in that moment, trust is not demanded—it begins to form.

The Emotional Mechanics: What the Patient Is Asking Without Saying It

Anger and distrust are rarely about the words being spoken. They are about questions that are *not* being spoken. Before the patient evaluates your explanation, your diagnosis, or your plan, they are asking something far more immediate:

- *Are you actually listening to me?*
- *Do I matter here?*
- *Are you going to dismiss me like others have?*

These questions are not asked directly. They are *felt*. And they are answered—quickly—by how you respond in the first moments.

A Dialogue Demonstration

Patient (frustrated, guarded):
I've been dealing with this for months. Every time I come in, I feel like nobody really hears what I'm saying.

What Happens If the Provider Moves Too Quickly to Explanation

Dr. Carter (focused on problem-solving**):**
"Let's go over your symptoms again and see what might be causing this."

(The patient withdraws slightly.)

The question *"Do I matter here?"* has not been answered.

The Correct Approach: Answer the Emotional Question First

Dr. Carter (calm, attentive):
It sounds like you've been feeling unheard throughout this process.

(Pause. Eye contact. No interruption.)

Patient (tone softens slightly):
Yeah… exactly.

What Just Happened

Before discussing symptoms, before offering solutions, the provider answered: *"Are you actually listening to me?"*

Going Deeper

Patient (more open now):
I just don't want to keep going through this and have it brushed off again.

Dr. Carter:
That makes sense.

(Pause.)

We're going to take this seriously and go through it carefully.

Now another question is answered: *"Do I matter here?"*

The Final Unspoken Question

Sometimes the most powerful one: *Are you going to dismiss me like others have?"*

The Provider Responds Without Saying It Directly

Dr. Carter:
Let's go through everything together, and I want to make sure we don't miss anything important.

(This is not just a plan—it is a reassurance of attention and respect.)

Why This Matters

If these emotional questions remain unanswered,

- the patient stays guarded,
- information is filtered through distrust, and
- even correct explanations are not fully received.

If they are answered early,

- the patient relaxes slightly,
- engagement increases, and
- the conversation becomes collaborative.

The Invisible Sequence

- The patient enters with emotion
- The provider responds
- The patient decides—often within seconds—"Am I safe to engage here?"

The Teaching Point

You are always answering two conversations at once:

- The *clinical conversation* (symptoms, diagnosis, plan)
- The *emotional conversation* (trust, safety, value)

If the second is ignored, the first is weakened.

The Principle to Remember

Your first response is not just about content; it is about connection. Before your explanation is heard, your presence is evaluated. And in that moment, the patient is not asking: *"What do you know?"* They are asking: "Are you here with me—or not?" When you answer that well, everything that follows becomes easier to receive.

What De-escalation Is Not

It is not:

1. Agreeing with everything the patient says
2. Avoiding difficult truths
3. Surrendering clinical judgment

What De-escalation Is: Moving from Reaction to Control

De-escalation is often misunderstood as simply *staying calm* or *being nice*. In reality, it is far more deliberate than that. It is an *active clinical skill*—one that requires control over your own responses while shaping the emotional direction of the encounter. You are not passively enduring the interaction.; you are *guiding it*.

Remaining Composed Under Pressure: Control of Self Before Control of Situation

When a patient is angry or distrustful, the pressure is immediate. The tone may feel personal. The words may feel unfair. Composure in this moment is not about suppressing reaction; it is about *choosing not to mirror the patient's state*.

Demonstration

Patient (sharp):
This whole process has been a mess. No one here knows what they're doing.

Provider (controlled, even tone):
I can hear how frustrating this has been.

What the provider resists:

- Matching tone
- Correcting immediately
- Defending competence

What the provider does instead:

- Slows the pace
- Keeps voice steady
- Maintains emotional neutrality

Why This Matters

The provider becomes the *emotional reference point* in the room. If you escalate, the patient escalates. If you remain steady, the interaction has a chance to stabilize.

Acknowledging the Patient's Experience Without Argument: Validation Without Agreement

Acknowledgment is not agreement. It is recognition.

Demonstration

Patient:
You people never follow up. I've been left in the dark.

Provider:
You've been waiting without clear communication, and that's been frustrating.

Notice the precision:

- The provider does not say, "You're right, we never follow up."
- The provider reflects the *experience*, not the accusation

Why This Matters

Argument creates opposition. Acknowledgment creates alignment. The patient no longer needs to prove their frustration; it has already been recognized.

Creating Structure Where There Is Emotional Chaos: Replacing Disorder with Direction

Anger and distrust are often disorganized states. The patient's thoughts jump. The concerns blur together. Structure brings order.

Demonstration

Provider:
Let's take this step by step.

(Pause.)

Here's what we know so far. Here's what we're still figuring out. And here's what we're doing next.

Why This Matters

Structure does three things immediately:

- Reduces overwhelm
- Clarifies the situation
- Reintroduces predictability

The patient shifts from reacting emotionally to following a process.

Redirecting Toward Clarity and Next Steps: From Emotion to Movement

De-escalation is not complete when the patient calms down. It is complete when the interaction moves forward constructively.

Demonstration

Patient (quieter now):
I just want to understand what's going on.

Provider:
Let's go through your results together, and then I'll outline exactly what happens next.

The provider does not stay in the emotional space indefinitely. They use stabilization as a bridge to clarity.

Why This Matters

Without redirection,

- the conversation circles around frustration, and
- no progress is made .

With redirection,

- the patient regains purpose, and
- the encounter becomes productive.

The Integration

True de-escalation is the combination of all four elements:

1. **Composure** keeps the interaction from worsening
2. **Acknowledgment** reduces resistance
3. **Structure** organizes the moment
4. **Direction** moves it forward

Remove any one of these, and the process weakens.

The Teaching Point

De-escalation is not about calming the patient down. It is about restoring conditions where care can continue.

The Principle to Remember

You are not absorbing emotion passively. You are transforming it from

- confrontation,
- distrust , and
- disorganization

to

- stability,
- alignment, and
- forward movement.

And when done correctly, the patient no longer feels the need to fight for control because they can feel that control has already been established.

De-escalation in Real Time: A Full Dialogue with Explanation

This is not a perfect patient. This is not a polite exchange. This is what it actually feels like when tension enters the room.

The Scenario

A patient arrives angry after a delayed diagnosis and multiple prior visits.

The Raw Interaction

Patient (immediately, voice raised):
This is unbelievable. I've been here three times, and nobody figured this out. Now, suddenly, it's serious? What have you people been doing?

What the Provider Does Not Do

There is no interruption. No correction. No defense.

Step 1: Composure

Dr. Harris (calm, steady, seated):
I can hear how upsetting this has been.

Explanation

This is the first turning point.

- The provider does not react emotionally
- The tone is slower than the patient's
- The statement reflects emotion, not facts

This prevents escalation.

Step 2: Acknowledgment Without Argument

Patient (still intense):
Of course it's upsetting. I trusted this place, and now I feel like everything was missed.

Dr. Harris:
You're feeling like something important wasn't caught when it should have been.

Explanation

Notice what is *not* said:

- No "we didn't miss anything"
- No "that's not accurate"

Instead, the provider translates the emotion into clear language. The patient feels understood, not opposed.

Step 3: Absorbing the Emotional Peak

Patient (voice still sharp, but less chaotic):
Exactly. And now I'm the one dealing with it.

Dr. Harris (slight nod):
That's a difficult place to be.

(Pause.)

Explanation

The pause matters as much as the words.

- It allows the patient's intensity to settle
- It shows the provider is not rushing to defend
- It creates space

Step 4: Introducing Structure

Dr. Harris (gently shifting):
Let's take this step by step so we can make sure you have a clear understanding of where things are now.

Explanation

This is the pivot. The provider moves from emotion to structure without skipping the emotional acknowledgment. Now the patient has something to follow.

Step 5: Redirecting Toward Clarity

Patient (quieter, but still guarded):
Alright… what does that even mean?

Dr. Harris:
Here's what we know right now.

(Pause.)

We've identified the issue, and we now have a clear plan to address it.

Explanation

The provider is not revisiting blame. They are reorienting toward current reality and forward movement.

Step 6: Restoring Partnership

Dr. Harris:
My focus right now is making sure you understand exactly what's happening and what we're doing next—and that we handle this carefully from here.

Patient (exhales, tone softer):
…I just don't want anything else missed.

Dr. Harris (steady):
Neither do I.

(Pause.)

That's why we're going to go through this thoroughly together.

Explanation

This is where the shift is completed. The patient moves from accusation to concern, and the provider aligns with that concern.

What Just Happened (Step-by-Step)

- **Composure prevented escalation:** The provider did not mirror anger.
- **Acknowledgment reduced resistance:** The patient no longer needed to argue to be heard.
- **Structure contained the emotion:** The conversation gained direction.
- **Redirection created forward movement:** Focus shifted from blame to a plan.

The Key Insight

At no point did the provider:

- Defend past care
- Argue facts
- Try to "win"

And yet, control of the interaction was never lost.

The Outcome

Patient (calmer now):
Okay… I just want to understand what we're doing.

That sentence is the goal: not agreement, not apology, but *engagement.*

The Principle to Remember

De-escalation is not about calming the patient by force. It is about

- absorbing intensity,
- organizing the moment, and
- guiding it forward.

When done correctly, the patient stops fighting the interaction and starts participating in it.

The Turning Point

The moment anger begins to soften is subtle. It often sounds like:

Patient (quieter):
I just want to understand what's going on.

At that point, the interaction shifts from confrontation to engagement.

The Teaching Point

You cannot control the patient's initial emotion. But you can control whether it escalates or settles.

The Principle to Remember

Do not meet anger with resistance. Do not meet distrust with authority. Meet both with

- calm acknowledgment,
- clear thinking, and
- transparent communication

Because when a patient feels heard—even briefly—they no longer need to raise their voice to be understood. And in that moment, the conversation becomes possible again.

Chapter 13

End-of-Life Conversations

Honesty, dignity, and presence

There are few moments in medicine more defining than the conversation in which a provider must acknowledge that time is no longer an abstract concept, but a finite and narrowing reality. End-of-life discussions are not simply clinical exchanges. They are deeply human encounters that sit at the intersection of truth, fear, hope, and meaning. In these moments, the provider is no longer just a provider of treatment, but a guide through one of life's most vulnerable transitions.

Honesty, in this context, is not bluntness. It is not the cold delivery of facts stripped of empathy. True honesty is measured, intentional, and compassionate. It requires the provider to communicate reality clearly, without removing the patient's sense of dignity or overwhelming them with despair. Patients often sense more than they are told. When information is withheld or softened to the point of distortion, trust begins to erode. The patient may feel isolated, as though they are navigating an unspoken truth alone. Honest communication, when done properly, does the opposite. It invites the patient into a shared understanding, allowing them to prepare, reflect, and make decisions that align with their values.

Dignity is preserved not through what is said, but how it is said and how the patient is treated throughout the conversation. A patient nearing the end of life is acutely aware of loss—loss of control, independence, identity, and future. The provider has the ability to restore a sense of agency by involving the patient in decisions, acknowledging their fears, and recognizing their life beyond the illness. Addressing a patient by name, sitting at eye level, allowing silence to exist without rushing to fill it—these are not small gestures. They communicate respect. They affirm that the patient is not defined by their diagnosis, but by their humanity.

Presence may be the most powerful element of all. In a medical culture often driven by efficiency and time constraints, the willingness to be fully present becomes rare—and therefore profoundly impactful. Presence is not about the duration of the conversation, but the quality of attention within it. It is the absence of distraction, the willingness to listen without interruption, and the ability to tolerate emotional discomfort without retreating into clinical detachment. Patients do not expect their providers to eliminate their fear. They expect them not to abandon them to it.

These conversations also require an understanding that hope does not disappear at the end of life; it simply changes form. Early in illness, hope may center around cure or prolonged survival. As the disease progresses, hope may shift toward comfort, reconciliation, meaningful time with loved ones, or a peaceful passing. A skilled provider does not extinguish hope but helps reshape it in a way that remains authentic. This reframing allows the patient to maintain a sense of purpose, even as outcomes become more limited.

Equally important is the recognition that end-of-life conversations are rarely a single event. They are an ongoing dialogue, evolving as the patient's condition and perspective change. What a patient is ready to hear today may differ from what they can process tomorrow. This requires patience, continuity, and emotional awareness. It also requires the provider to read not only what is spoken, but what is avoided—the pauses, the hesitations, the questions that are asked indirectly.

Family dynamics often enter the space as well, adding complexity. Loved ones may seek protection from the truth, while the patient may desire clarity. Or the reverse may be true. Navigating these differences requires balance. The provider must remain anchored to the patient's autonomy while maintaining compassion for the emotional responses of those around them. This is not a negotiation of facts, but a careful alignment of communication with the patient's expressed wishes.

There is also a subtle but critical distinction between delivering information and creating understanding. A provider can state that a condition is terminal, yet fail to ensure the patient truly grasps what that means for their time, choices, and priorities. Understanding emerges through dialogue, through checking for comprehension, and through allowing space for questions that may not come immediately. Silence, in these moments, is not a void. It is often where the most important processing occurs.

For the provider, these conversations can be emotionally demanding. There is a natural inclination to avoid discomfort, to redirect toward treatment options, or to maintain distance as a form of self-protection. However, it is within this discomfort that the most meaningful care is often delivered. The ability to remain steady, to neither withdraw nor overcompensate, reflects a level of professional maturity that cannot be taught solely through textbooks. It is developed through reflection, experience, and an ongoing commitment to seeing patients as individuals rather than cases.

Ultimately, end-of-life conversations are not about death alone. They are about how a person is seen, heard, and supported in the final chapter of their life. When handled with honesty, dignity, and presence, these moments can transform from something feared into something profoundly meaningful. They allow patients to retain control over their narrative, to find closure where possible, and to face the unknown with a sense that they are not alone.

In the broader scope of medicine, these conversations reveal a fundamental truth: the role of the provider is not only to extend life when possible, but to honor it fully when it cannot be prolonged.

Within end-of-life care, the most meaningful conversations are not defined by their medical content, but by their depth of human truth. They move beyond diagnosis and prognosis into identity, meaning, fear, and closure. In each of these, the provider's role quietly shifts from expert to guide, from problem-solver to witness.

"Am I dying?" — The Conversation of Reality

This is often the most direct and most feared question. It is rarely just about medical confirmation; it is about whether the patient can trust you with the truth. The provider's role is to answer with clarity and compassion, avoiding both evasion and bluntness. This is where honesty must be calibrated. The goal is not simply to inform, but to anchor the patient in reality without stripping them of their emotional footing. The provider becomes a stabilizing presence in a moment where the ground feels as though it is shifting.

Provider:
I want to sit with you for a moment, without rushing. How are you feeling today?

Patient:
Tired… but more than that, uncertain. I feel like something has changed.

Provider:
I hear that. Can you tell me what feels different?

Patient:
It feels like time is shorter… like we're not talking about getting better anymore.

Provider:
You're right to sense that. The illness has reached a point where our focus is shifting.

Patient:
Shifting… meaning I'm dying?

Provider:
Yes. And I want to walk through this with you, honestly and gently.

Patient:
I appreciate you saying it plainly. How much time do I have?

Provider:
I can't give an exact number, but I believe we are talking in terms of months, not years.

Patient:
Months… that's hard to hear.

Provider:
I understand. Take your time. I'm here with you.

Patient:
What will it be like? Will I be in pain?

Provider:
Our priority will be your comfort. We have ways to manage pain and keep you as peaceful as possible.

Patient:
I don't want to suffer… or lose myself completely.

Provider:
We will do everything we can to preserve your comfort and your dignity. That matters deeply.

Patient:
What choices do I have now?

Provider:
You can continue treatments, or we can focus fully on comfort and quality of life, possibly with hospice support.

Patient:
Choosing comfort… that's not giving up?

Provider:
Not at all. It's choosing how you want to live the time you have.

Patient:
I think… I want to be at home, with my family.

Provider:
That's something we can absolutely help arrange.

Patient:
I worry about being a burden to them.

Provider:
It's natural to feel that way. But being cared for is not the same as being a burden. You matter to them.

Patient:
I hope they know how much they mean to me.

Provider:
There is still time to say those things, in your own way.

Patient:
Will you… still be here through this?

Provider:
Yes. I will not step away. We will face this together.

Patient:
That helps more than you know.

Provider:
You don't have to carry this alone.

"How much time do I have?" — The Conversation of Uncertainty

Time, in these moments, becomes deeply personal. Patients are not only asking for a number; they are asking how to think about the time that remains. The provider's role is to frame uncertainty honestly while still offering guidance. Rather than rigid timelines, the provider helps the patient understand ranges, possibilities, and what to expect functionally. This transforms time from a countdown into something the patient can still shape.

Provider:
You've been quiet today. What's on your mind?

Patient:
I keep thinking about one thing… and I don't know how to ask it.

Provider:
You can ask me anything. Take your time.

Patient:
How much time do I have?

Provider:
That's an important question. Can you tell me what's making you ask it right now?

Patient:
I feel things changing. I get weaker. I can't do what I could even a few weeks ago. I need to understand what I'm facing.

Provider:
I hear you. And I want to be honest with you, while also being careful not to give you a false sense of certainty.

Patient:
I don't need exact… I just need something real.

Provider:
Based on what we're seeing, I would think in terms of months rather than years. But within that, there is still uncertainty.

Patient:
Months… that's hard, but I expected it. What will those months be like?

Provider:
That's the more important question. You may notice increasing fatigue, needing more help with daily activities, and spending more time resting. But we will focus on keeping you comfortable.

Patient:
Will I still have time where I feel like myself?

Provider:
Yes. There can still be meaningful, clear moments. Time with family, conversations, quiet experiences that matter.

Patient:
I don't want to just count down the days.

Provider:
And you don't have to. This isn't only about how long, but about how that time is lived.

Patient:
I think… I want to use that time differently now.

Provider:
That's something we can plan for. What feels most important to you?

Patient:
Being at home. Talking to my family. Not being in and out of hospitals.

Provider:
Those are clear priorities. We can align your care to support exactly that.

Patient:
So even if I can't control how long… I can still shape what's left?

Provider:
Yes. You still have that control. That matters.

Patient:
Thank you for not avoiding the question.

Provider:
You deserve honesty, and you deserve guidance through it.

Patient:
I feel scared… but also a little clearer.

Provider:
That's okay. We can hold both of those feelings together.

Patient:
Will you help me through what comes next?

Provider:
I will be here with you, every step of the way.

"What will happen to me?" — The Conversation of Fear

Here, the patient is asking about suffering, loss of control, and the process of dying itself. Often, this question is layered with unspoken fears of pain, dependence, or being a burden. The provider's role is to demystify the process. By explaining what is likely to occur and how symptoms will be managed, fear becomes more defined and therefore more manageable. The provider becomes a translator of the unknown into something that can be faced.

Provider:
You seem a little unsettled today. What's weighing on you?

Patient:
I keep thinking about what's coming… and I can't stop.

Provider:
Tell me what you're imagining.

Patient:
I don't know exactly. I just… what will happen to me?

Provider:
That's a very real and important question. When you ask that, what worries you the most?

Patient:
Pain. Losing control. Not being myself. Maybe… being a burden to everyone.

Provider:
Those are very common fears, and I'm glad you said them out loud. Let's talk through each of them together.

Patient:
I just don't want to suffer.

Provider:
Our primary goal will be your comfort. We have very effective ways to manage pain, shortness of breath, and anxiety. You will not be left to suffer.

Patient:
And losing control? That scares me too.

Provider:
You may notice gradual changes. More fatigue, needing help with daily things. But we will involve you in decisions as long as possible, and we will respect your wishes throughout.

Patient:
Will I know what's happening? Or will I just… fade?

Provider:
Many patients remain aware for much of the time. As the body slows down, there is often more sleep, less awareness, and a natural quieting. It is usually not sudden or chaotic.

Patient:
That sounds… calmer than I imagined.

Provider:
That's important to understand. What people fear is often much harsher than what actually occurs, especially with proper care.

Patient:
I don't want my family to see me like that.

Provider:
It's natural to feel that way. But families often don't see burden—they see love and the opportunity to be present with you.

Patient:
I never thought of it that way.

Provider:
You're still you, through all of this. That doesn't disappear.

Patient:
I think part of me was afraid to even ask.

Provider:
And yet asking is what makes it less frightening. The unknown is always heavier when it's unspoken.

Patient:
It feels a little more… manageable now.

Provider:
That's the goal. Not to remove all fear, but to make it something you don't have to face alone or in the dark.

Patient:
Will you help guide me through it?

Provider:
Yes. I will be here to explain, to support, and to make sure you are as comfortable and cared for as possible.

Patient:
Thank you… that means more than I can say.

Provider:
You don't have to go through this without understanding. We will face it together.

"What are my options?" — The Conversation of Control

At the end of life, control often feels like it is slipping away. This question is an attempt to reclaim some agency. The provider's role is to present choices clearly and without bias—continuing treatment, shifting to comfort-focused care, hospice, or other pathways. More importantly, the provider ensures the patient understands that choosing comfort is not "giving up," but an active, values-based decision. The provider becomes an advocate for the patient's autonomy.

Provider:
We've talked about where things are medically. I want to make sure we also talk about what comes next—on your terms.

Patient:
That's what I've been thinking about. What are my options?

Provider:
You do have options, and it's important that you understand them clearly so you can decide what feels right to you.

Patient:
I don't want to feel like things are just happening to me.

Provider:
And they don't have to. You still have a voice in how this unfolds.

Patient:
So… what can I choose?

Provider:
One option is to continue treatments aimed at slowing the illness, knowing they may come with side effects and time in the hospital.

Patient:
And the other?

Provider:
Another option is to shift the focus entirely to comfort—managing symptoms, reducing hospital visits, and prioritizing quality of life.

Patient:
That's hospice?

Provider:
Hospice is one form of that approach. It provides support at home or in a comfortable setting, focusing on you rather than the disease.

Patient:
Choosing that… it feels like giving up.

Provider:
I understand why it can feel that way. But it's not giving up. It's choosing what matters most to you with the time you have.

Patient:
So, it's still a decision… not a surrender.

Provider:
Exactly. It's an active, thoughtful choice based on your values.

Patient:
What would you recommend?

Provider:
My role is to guide you, not to decide for you. What matters most is what feels meaningful and right in your life.

Patient:
I think I value being comfortable… being with my family… more than more treatments.

Provider:
That clarity is important. We can shape your care around those priorities.

Patient:
And if I change my mind?

Provider:
You can. These decisions are not locked in. We can adjust as your needs and feelings evolve.

Patient:
That helps. I was afraid of making the wrong choice.

Provider:
There isn't a "right" or "wrong" here—only what aligns with who you are and what you want.

Patient:
I just want to feel like I still have some control.

Provider:
You do. And I'm here to protect that, every step of the way.

Patient:
Thank you for explaining it this way.

Provider:
You deserve to understand your options—and to choose your path with clarity and dignity.

"What matters most to me now?" — The Conversation of Meaning

This is rarely asked directly, but it is often the most important conversation. It may emerge through statements about family, unfinished goals, or personal values. The provider's role is to help the patient articulate these priorities and align care accordingly. This may mean facilitating time at home, enabling meaningful interactions, or avoiding interventions that would detract from quality of life. The provider becomes a listener who helps define what a "good ending" means for that individual.

Provider:
We've talked about the medical side of things. I'd like to understand something more personal, if that's okay.

Patient:
What do you mean?

Provider:
Given everything that's happening… what feels most important to you right now?

Patient:
I'm not sure I've thought about it that way.

Provider:
That's alright. Sometimes it's not a question we ask ourselves directly. We can take it slowly.

Patient:
I guess… I keep thinking about my family.

Provider:
Tell me more about that.

Patient:
I don't want to spend whatever time I have left in hospitals. I want to be with them… at home.

Provider:
Being at home, surrounded by the people you love—that sounds like a priority.

Patient:
Yes. I want things to feel normal, as much as they can.

Provider:
That's something we can help make possible by shaping your care around that goal.

Patient:
I also feel like there are things I haven't said yet.

Provider:
Important things?

Patient:
Very. Conversations I've put off… things I want them to know.

Provider:
Having the space and clarity for those conversations can be one of the most meaningful parts of this time.

Patient:
I don't want to be too weak or too out of it to say them.

Provider:
Then we can focus on preserving your energy and minimizing interventions that might take that away from you.

Patient:
That matters more to me than anything else right now.

Provider:
What you're describing is a clear sense of what gives your time meaning.

Patient:
I think I'm starting to see that. It's not about how long… it's about what I do with it.

Provider:
Exactly. And my role is to help align your care with those priorities.

Patient:
So, choosing less treatment might actually give me more of what I want?

Provider:
In many cases, yes. It allows your time to be spent where and how it matters most to you.

Patient:
I want to be present… not just alive.

Provider:
That distinction is very important, and we can honor it.

Patient:
I'm glad you asked me this. I didn't realize how much I needed to think about it.

Provider:
These conversations often reveal what truly matters.

Patient:
I feel clearer now. Like I have direction.

Provider:
And that clarity helps us support you in a way that reflects your life, not just your illness.

Patient:
Thank you for listening… really listening.

Provider:
It's a privilege to understand what matters most to you.

"Will I be a burden?" — The Conversation of Worth

Many patients carry a quiet fear that their illness imposes too much on those they love. This question is often expressed indirectly. The provider's role is to acknowledge this concern without dismissing it, while reinforcing the patient's inherent value. By involving support systems, palliative care, and realistic planning, the provider helps reframe the patient not as a burden, but as a person still deserving of care and presence.

Provider:
You've been thoughtful today. What's been on your mind?

Patient:
I haven't said this out loud yet… but I keep thinking about it.

Provider:
You can say anything here.

Patient:
I don't want to become a burden to my family.

Provider:
That's a very real concern, and many people feel that way. Tell me what that looks like in your mind.

Patient:
Needing help with everything… them having to watch me decline… putting their lives on hold because of me.

Provider:
It sounds like you're worried not just about yourself, but about the weight this might place on them.

Patient:
Exactly. I don't want my last chapter to be something that harms them.

Provider:
I understand that. But I want you to hear something clearly—you are not a burden. You are someone they love.

Patient:
It doesn't always feel that way.

Provider:
That feeling often comes from a place of care, not reality. Love changes how people experience responsibility.

Patient:
But it's still hard on them, isn't it?

Provider:
It can be difficult, yes. But difficulty and burden are not the same. Being present for someone they love often holds deep meaning for them.

Patient:
I never thought of it like that.

Provider:
We can also put support in place—palliative care, hospice teams, resources that help share the responsibility, so it doesn't fall entirely on your family.

Patient:
So, they won't be alone in this either?

Provider:
Exactly. You will be supported, and so will they.

Patient:
I just don't want to lose my sense of worth.

Provider:
Your worth is not defined by what you can do physically. It's defined by who you are, and that does not change.

Patient:
It's hard to hold on to that when everything else is changing.

Provider:
That's why these conversations matter. To remind you that your value remains constant, even as circumstances shift.

Patient:
I still want to give something to them… not just take.

Provider:
Your presence, your words, your connection—those are things only you can give. And they matter deeply.

Patient:
I suppose being there with them still counts for something.

Provider:
It counts for more than you may realize.

Patient:
I feel a little lighter saying this out loud.

Provider:
Sometimes naming the fear is what begins to loosen its hold.

Patient:
Thank you for not brushing it aside.

Provider:
It deserves to be heard, and so do you.

"What happens after I'm gone?" — The Conversation of Legacy

This can take many forms: concerns about family, unresolved relationships, or how one will be remembered. The provider's role is not to provide answers to existential unknowns, but to create space for these reflections. Sometimes this includes encouraging conversations with loved ones, addressing unfinished emotional matters, or simply witnessing the patient's thoughts without redirecting them back to medicine. The provider becomes a quiet participant in the patient's search for closure.

Provider:
You seem reflective today. What's been on your mind?

Patient:
I've been thinking about something I haven't said before.

Provider:
You can share it, whenever you're ready.

Patient:
What happens… after I'm gone?

Provider:
That question can mean many things. What does it mean to you?

Patient:
My family… what their lives will look like. If they'll be okay. If they'll remember me the right way.

Provider:
It sounds like you're thinking about the impact you leave behind.

Patient:
Yes. I don't want to just disappear. I want to feel like something of me stays with them.

Provider:
In many ways, it already does. Through your relationships, your influence, your presence in their lives.

Patient:
I hope so. I worry about things I didn't finish… things I didn't say.

Provider:
Those things can still be addressed. There is time to speak, to write, to connect in ways that feel meaningful to you.

Patient:
I wouldn't even know where to start.

Provider:
Sometimes it begins with something simple, telling someone what they've meant to you, or what you hope for them.

Patient:
I'd like them to remember me with peace… not sadness.

Provider:
Sharing that with them can shape how they carry you forward.

Patient:
Do people really hold on to those moments?

Provider:
Very much so. Often, it's those words and connections that stay with them the longest.

Patient:
I think there are things I need to say to my son… things I've avoided.

Provider:
This could be an opportunity to say them in a way that brings clarity and closure—for both of you.

Patient:
I don't want to leave things unresolved.

Provider:
Wanting resolution is a powerful and human instinct. And it's something you can still move toward.

Patient:
I always thought legacy meant something big… but maybe it's more personal than that.

Provider:
Often, it is. It lives in relationships, in memories, in the way you've shaped the people around you.

Patient:
That makes it feel more real… and more within reach.

Provider:
It is within reach. And I'm here to support you as you think through what matters most to leave behind.

Patient:
Thank you for not turning this into something clinical.

Provider:
Some questions aren't meant to be answered with medicine—they're meant to be heard.

Patient:
I'm glad I said it out loud.

Provider:
I'm glad you did too.

Silence: The Conversation Without Words

At times, the deepest exchange is not verbal at all. A pause, a tear, a moment of stillness can carry more meaning than any explanation. The provider's role here is restraint. Not to fill the silence, not to retreat from it, but to remain present within it. This requires comfort with discomfort and a willingness to let the patient lead the emotional pace.

Across all of these conversations, the provider's role is unified by three underlying responsibilities:

- To tell the truth without causing harm,
- to preserve dignity when it feels most threatened, and
- to remain present when there is nothing left to fix.

In this space, the provider is no longer measured solely by knowledge or technical skill, but by their ability to stand alongside another human being at the edge of life—and not look away.

Part IV

The Healthcare Provider's Internal World

Chapter 14	Emotional Detachment vs. Emotional Control	194
Chapter 15	Burnout and Its Effect on Communication	201
Chapter 16	Time Pressure and Its Consequences	205
Chapter 17	Maintaining Humanity in a System That Demands Efficiency	210

Chapter 14

Emotional Detachment vs. Emotional Control

The Difference That Defines Good Care

In healthcare, emotional balance is often misunderstood. Many professionals are taught—explicitly or implicitly—that detachment is necessary to survive the demands of the job. Over time, this belief can evolve into a quiet but dangerous habit: distancing oneself emotionally from patients in order to function efficiently. While this may protect the provider in the short term, it often erodes the very foundation of meaningful care.

There is, however, a critical distinction that separates average care from exceptional care: emotional *detachment* vs. *emotional control.*

Emotional Detachment: The Quiet Disconnect

Emotional detachment occurs when a provider unconsciously or deliberately creates distance from a patient's experience. It may show up as:

- Minimal eye contact
- Rushed or transactional communication
- Avoidance of emotionally charged conversations
- A focus on diagnosis over the person

At its core, detachment is a *protective mechanism*—a way to avoid feeling overwhelmed. But the unintended consequence is that patients feel unseen, unheard, and reduced to a condition rather than recognized as a person.

Detached care may be clinically accurate, but it is often *emotionally insufficient*. Patients can sense when a provider is disengaged. Trust weakens. Compliance may drop. And most importantly, the healing relationship—the one that can influence outcomes just as much as treatment—is compromised.

Emotional Control: The Skilled Presence

Emotional control, by contrast, is not about shutting down feelings—it is about *managing them effectively while remaining fully present.* A provider practicing emotional control:

- Acknowledges emotions without being overwhelmed by them
- Maintains composure in high-stress situations
- Demonstrates empathy without losing clinical clarity
- Stays engaged, attentive, and human

This is not an easy balance. It requires awareness, discipline, and practice. But it is the hallmark of high-quality care. Emotionally controlled providers do not withdraw—they *lean in with intention.* They understand that emotions are not liabilities; they are tools. When managed properly, they enhance communication, strengthen trust, and deepen patient connection.

Why This Difference Matters

The distinction between detachment and control is subtle but powerful:

- Detachment protects the provider but distances the patient
- Control protects both the provider and the relationship

In moments of vulnerability—receiving a diagnosis, facing uncertainty, dealing with pain—patients are not just seeking answers. They are seeking reassurance, understanding, and connection. A provider who is emotionally controlled can say, through both words and presence: "I see you. I hear you. And I'm here with you." That message alone can change the entire care experience.

Dialogue 1: The Detached Encounter

Patient:
I've been really worried about these results… I haven't been sleeping.

Provider (looking at computer):
Well, your labs show elevated levels. We'll start you on medication.

Patient:
Is it serious?

Provider:
It's manageable. Just follow the prescription.

Patient (hesitant):
I just… feel overwhelmed.

Provider (standing up):
Schedule a follow-up in four weeks.

Analysis: The provider is efficient but emotionally absent. The patient's fear is acknowledged only indirectly, leaving them feeling alone and uncertain.

Dialogue 2: Emotional Overload (Lack of Control)

Patient:
I'm scared. My father had the same condition… and it didn't end well.

Provider (visibly tense):
I know… it's really hard. Cases like this can be very difficult.

Patient:
So… does that mean the same thing will happen to me?

Provider (voice soft, uncertain):
I… I don't want to say that, but… it's possible.

Patient (distressed):
I don't know how to handle this.

Provider:
I understand… it's a lot.

Analysis: Here, the provider is emotionally engaged but lacks control. Their anxiety transfers to the patient, increasing fear rather than stabilizing it.

Dialogue 3: Emotionally Controlled Care

Patient:
I'm really scared. My father had this, and it didn't go well.

Provider (making eye contact):
I hear how much that's weighing on you. Anyone in your position would feel that way.

Patient:
So… is this going to happen to me too?

Provider (calm, steady):
Your situation is not the same as your father's. We've caught this early, and we have effective ways to manage it.

Patient (exhaling slightly):
Okay… that helps a little.

Provider:
We're going to take this step by step, together. You won't have to navigate this alone.

Analysis: The provider acknowledges emotion without absorbing it. They remain calm, grounded, and reassuring—creating safety while maintaining clinical clarity.

The Defining Standard of Care

Great healthcare is not defined solely by knowledge or technical skill. It is defined by the ability to remain human under pressure.

- Not cold, but not overwhelmed
- Not distant, but not consumed
- Not detached, but in control

Emotional control allows providers to build trust without burning out, to connect without losing clarity, and to care deeply without losing themselves. This is the difference patients remember. This is the difference that defines good care.

The Provider's Hidden Barrier: Fear of Becoming Emotional

One of the least discussed—but most influential—barriers to meaningful patient care is not clinical workload, time pressure, or system constraints. It is the provider's internal fear of becoming emotional. This fear often goes unrecognized. It hides beneath professionalism, efficiency, and the belief that "staying objective" requires emotional distance. But in reality, many providers are not choosing detachment because it is best for the patient—they are choosing it because it feels safer for themselves.

Understanding the Fear

Healthcare providers are repeatedly exposed to:

- Suffering
- Uncertainty
- Loss
- High-stakes decisions

Over time, this creates a subconscious concern: "If I allow myself to feel too much, I may lose control." This fear can take several forms:

- Fear of breaking down in front of a patient
- Fear of saying the wrong thing emotionally
- Fear of becoming too attached and being hurt
- Fear that empathy will interfere with clinical judgment

These are not weaknesses—they are human responses to intense environments. But when left unexamined, they quietly shape behavior.

The Problem: Fear Leads to Avoidance

When providers fear their own emotional responses, they often compensate by:

- Keeping conversations strictly clinical
- Redirecting emotional expressions quickly

- Limiting time spent with vulnerable patients
- Creating subtle interpersonal distance

This is not intentional neglect—it is *emotional self-protection*. However, patients experience this as indifference.

The Shift: From Fear to Mastery

The goal is not to eliminate emotion. That is neither realistic nor desirable. The goal is to build confidence in one's ability to handle emotion without being controlled by it. In other words, the issue is not emotion itself—the issue is the provider's belief that emotion is unmanageable.

When providers develop emotional control, something powerful happens:

- Fear decreases
- Presence increases
- Communication improves
- Burnout risk may actually decline (because suppression is exhausting)

Reframing Emotional Exposure

Instead of viewing emotion as a threat, providers can begin to see it as:

- **Information**: What is this patient feeling? What do they need right now?
- **Connection:** This is where trust is built
- **Opportunity:** This is often the moment that defines the care experience

Emotional moments are not interruptions to care—they are central to care.

Practical Internal Work for Providers

To move from fear to control, providers must engage in intentional self-awareness:

1. Recognize the trigger

Notice when you feel the urge to withdraw or shut down. That moment is often driven by discomfort, not necessity.

2. Name the fear internally

A simple internal acknowledgment (*"I'm worried I might get too emotional here"*) can reduce its power.

3. Separate feeling from action

You can feel empathy without losing composure. Feeling does not equal losing control.

4. Practice staying present for a few seconds longer

Often, growth happens in small increments—maintaining eye contact, allowing silence, or acknowledging emotion before moving on.

5. Reflect After Encounters

Instead of avoiding emotional cases, revisit them mentally:

- What did I feel?
- What did I avoid?
- What could I handle next time?

A Defining Realization

Many providers operate under this assumption: "If I open the door to emotion, I won't be able to close it." But experience shows the opposite is true: The more you practice managing emotion, the more control you gain over it. Avoidance preserves fear. Engagement builds skill.

Dialogue: Confronting the Fear Internally

(Internal dialogue — Provider before entering room)

Provider:
This patient just got bad news… I don't want this to get too emotional.

Pause

Provider (*reframing*):
Okay. I might feel something—and that's fine. I don't need to avoid it. I just need to stay steady.

(Inside the room)

Patient:
I don't even know how to process this…

Provider (*grounded, present***)**:
I can see how heavy this feels. We can take this one step at a time.

The Outcome

The provider did not suppress emotion. They did not lose control. They managed their internal fear, allowing them to show up fully.

The Core Truth

The greatest barrier to emotional control is not emotion itself—it is *fear of emotion*. When providers address this fear directly, they unlock a higher level of care:

- More authentic
- More connected
- More effective

And ultimately, more human.

Closing Reflection

The question is not: "How do I avoid becoming emotional?" The better question is: "Can I trust myself to handle emotion when it arises?" That trust—once developed—is what separates guarded providers from truly present ones. And it is often the difference patients feel most.

Chapter 15

Burnout and Its Effect on Communication

When Exhaustion Becomes Visible

Burnout in medicine rarely announces itself in dramatic fashion. It does not begin with collapse. It begins quietly, almost imperceptibly, in the subtle erosion of presence. The provider is still there, still functioning, still making decisions. But something essential has thinned.

And patients can feel it.

Not because the provider says the wrong words, but because the *space around the words has changed.* Communication, at its highest level, is not simply the exchange of information. It is the transmission of attention, steadiness, and intent. Burnout disrupts all three.

Before Burnout (Presence Intact)

Patient:
I've been feeling really tired... more than usual. I don't know, something just feels off.

Provider:
Tell me more about that. When you say 'off,' what does that feel like for you?

Patient:
It's hard to explain. I'm sleeping, but I wake up exhausted.

Provider:
That sounds frustrating. Let's slow this down and look at it together—your sleep, your stress, and anything else that might be contributing.

Patient:
Okay... I appreciate that.

(The patient feels engaged. The room feels unhurried. There is space to think.)

During Burnout (Exhaustion Becoming Visible)

Patient:
I've been feeling really tired… more than usual. I don't know, something just feels off.

Provider:
How many hours are you sleeping?

Patient:
About seven, maybe eight.

Provider:
Any recent illness? Changes in diet?

Patient:
No… not really.

Provider:
Okay. We can run some labs to check for common causes.

Patient:
…Alright.

(The information is gathered. The plan is appropriate. But something is missing.)

What the Patient Feels but Cannot Easily Name

In both conversations, the provider is competent. Nothing incorrect is said. No steps are missed. And yet:

- In the first, the provider is *with* the patient
- In the second, the provider is *processing* the patient

The difference is not in the words themselves, but in what surrounds them:

- The absence of pause
- The narrowing of curiosity
- The shift from exploration to checklist

Where Burnout Reveals Itself

It reveals itself in small ways.

Patient:
I don't know… I just feel like something's wrong.

Provider (burnout present):
We'll check your labs.

Provider (presence intact):
Let's take a moment and understand what 'wrong' feels like to you.

The burned-out provider has not stopped caring. But their capacity to stay present long enough to show it has been reduced. And patients, even without medical knowledge, are exquisitely sensitive to that difference. They may leave with answers, but not always with reassurance. They may receive care, but not always feel cared for. That is how burnout becomes visible: not in what is said, but in what is no longer felt.

The first shift is often *compression.* Conversations become shorter, more transactional. Questions are answered but not explored. The provider begins to anticipate rather than listen, to conclude rather than remain curious. Efficiency quietly replaces engagement.

The second shift is *emotional narrowing.* Where there was once a range of responsiveness, there is now a flattening. Not coldness, exactly—but a reduced ability to meet the patient where they are. Empathy becomes effortful. Silence becomes uncomfortable. The provider may still say the right phrases, but they are delivered without depth. Patients sense this immediately. They may not articulate it, but they feel less seen.

The third shift is *irritability at the margins.* Small interruptions feel larger. Repeated questions feel heavier. The provider's threshold for frustration lowers, not because they care less, but because they have less reserve from which to draw. What once would have been absorbed with ease now creates internal strain and occasionally visible impatience.

And this is where burnout becomes most evident: not in clinical error, but in *relational fracture.*

A Brief Clinical Contrast

Before burnout:

Patient:
I know you already explained it, but I'm still confused...

Provider:
That's completely okay. Let's go through it again—this time a little differently.

During burnout:

Patient:
I know you already explained it, but I'm still confused...

Provider:
I just went over that. It's in your discharge paperwork.

Both responses are factually acceptable. Only one preserves the relationship. Burnout does not eliminate skill. It alters *how that skill is delivered.*

A burned-out provider may still diagnose correctly, prescribe appropriately, and document thoroughly. But the patient experiences something different: a subtle sense of distance, a lack of ease, a feeling that their presence is one more task to be completed rather than a person to be understood.

This has consequences beyond satisfaction. Communication under strain becomes less adaptive. Important details may be missed, not from lack of knowledge, but from reduced attentional bandwidth. Patients may withhold concerns if they perceive the provider as rushed or unavailable. Trust, once fractured in small ways, becomes harder to build in larger ones.

The Paradox of Burnout

What makes burnout particularly complex is that it often affects those who care the most. The same individuals who once extended themselves fully begin to retract—not out of indifference, but out of necessity. Burnout is, in many ways, a protective adaptation. It creates distance to preserve function. But in doing so, it compromises the very connection that defines meaningful care.

When Exhaustion Becomes Visible

It becomes visible in tone, in pacing, and in the absence of small but significant pauses. It appears when the provider no longer has the margin to notice—the hesitation before a patient speaks, the uncertainty behind a question, the emotion behind a symptom. And yet, awareness of this process is itself powerful. Because the goal is not to demand constant emotional availability. That is neither realistic nor sustainable. The goal is more precise: to recognize when exhaustion is shaping communication, and to restore, even briefly, a deliberate sense of presence. Sometimes this is not a grand intervention. It is a single moment of recalibration:

- A breath before responding
- A decision to sit rather than stand
- A sentence that acknowledges rather than redirects

Burnout does not mean a provider has failed. But unrecognized burnout quietly reshapes how care is experienced. And in medicine, how something is experienced is never separate from what is delivered.

Chapter 16

Time Pressure and Its Consequences

Why Rushed Care Feels Like Careless Care

Time pressure in medicine is often framed as a logistical problem, a matter of scheduling, volume, and efficiency. But at the level of human experience, it becomes something far more consequential. It reshapes how care is delivered, and more importantly, how it is perceived.

A rushed encounter rarely feels neutral to a patient. It feels personal. Not because the provider intends it that way, but because patients interpret time as a signal of value. The amount of attention they receive becomes, in their minds, a reflection of how seriously they are being taken. When time is compressed, presence is often the first casualty. The provider may still ask the necessary questions, perform the appropriate exam, and arrive at a correct plan. Yet the interaction feels abbreviated, and with that, something essential is lost.

Patients begin to sense that the provider is moving ahead of them rather than with them. This creates a subtle but important shift. The patient speaks, but more cautiously. They may omit details, sensing there is little room for elaboration. Questions go unasked, not because they are unimportant, but because they feel inconvenient. The encounter becomes efficient, but incomplete.

Here is a dialogue that reveals both the spoken exchange and the patient's internal experience, where time pressure quietly reshapes the interaction:

Clinical Encounter Under Time Pressure

Provider:
Good morning. What brings you in today?

Patient:
I've been having some stomach pain… on and off for a few weeks.
Okay, just say the main thing. Don't take too long.

Provider:
Where exactly is the pain?

Patient:
Mostly upper abdomen… sometimes after I eat.
Should I mention the weight loss? Maybe later.

Provider:
Any nausea or vomiting?

Patient:
A little nausea, yes.

Provider:
Any medications? Alcohol use?

Patient:
No medications. I drink occasionally.
He's moving fast… maybe this is routine.

Provider:
Alright. This sounds like it could be gastritis or reflux. I'll start you on medication and we'll see how you respond.

Patient:
Okay…
That was quick… is that enough to know?

Provider:
Take this for a few weeks. If it doesn't improve, follow up.

Patient:
Alright, thank you.
I guess that's it. Maybe I'm overthinking it.

What Remains Unsaid

(Patient leaves the room)

Patient:
I never mentioned the weight loss, or that the pain wakes me up at night. He didn't ask, and he seemed in a hurry. It's probably nothing… but what if it's not?

What Just Happened

Nothing in the dialogue is incorrect. The provider asked appropriate questions. A reasonable plan was made. And yet:

- The patient filtered themselves
- Important details were withheld
- Uncertainty remained unspoken

Not because the patient was unwilling, but because the interaction signaled: "Keep this brief."

Why It Feels Personal

From the provider's perspective, the visit was efficient. From the patient's perspective:

- The pace felt like pressure
- The brevity felt like disinterest
- The lack of pause felt like a lack of concern

The provider moved forward. The patient held back.

The Quiet Consequence

Rushed care does not just shorten conversations. It reshapes them. Patients begin to edit themselves in real time, asking not, *"What do I need to say?"* but rather, *"What is worth saying here?"* And in that shift, care becomes incomplete—not because of what was done, but because of what was never allowed to surface.

A Brief Clinical Contrast

Patient:
I've also been having this tight feeling in my chest sometimes...

Provider:
Is it with exertion?

Patient:
Not always...

Provider:
Okay, we'll note that. Let's focus on your main concern today.

(The visit stays on track. But something potentially important has been sidelined.)

With preserved presence, even under constraint:

Patient:
I've also been having this tight feeling in my chest sometimes...

Provider:
I'm glad you mentioned that. Even briefly, I want to understand it—when it happens and what it feels like. We'll make sure it doesn't get overlooked.

(The time may still be limited. But the patient feels that what they said mattered.)

The difference is not always measured in minutes. It is measured in *attention*. A provider under time pressure often begins to prioritize completion over exploration. This is not a failure of character, but a response to system demands. However, patients do not experience the system. They experience the interaction. And when that interaction feels hurried, it can easily be interpreted as disinterest or dismissal.

This is where rushed care begins to resemble careless care. Not because the provider is careless, but because the patient no longer feels carefully held within the encounter.

The Hidden Consequences

When time pressure consistently shapes communication:

- Patients become less forthcoming
- Providers receive less complete information
- Misunderstandings increase
- Trust becomes more fragile

Over time, this can subtly erode the quality of care, even when clinical decisions remain sound.

A More Precise Understanding

Time pressure does not eliminate the ability to connect. But it demands *intentionality*: a brief pause, a sentence that acknowledges, a moment that signals, *"I am here, even if time is limited."* These are small adjustments, but they recalibrate the entire interaction. Because in the end, patients are not measuring the clock. They are measuring whether, within that time, they were seen, heard, and taken seriously. And when that is missing, even excellent care can feel insufficient.

Here is a dialogue that demonstrates how intentional presence—even under time pressure—changes the entire experience:

Clinical Encounter: Limited Time, Preserved Connection

Provider (glancing at chart, then pausing before speaking):
Good morning. I know we have a limited visit today, but I want to make sure we focus on what matters most to you.

Patient:
He's busy… but he said that directly. Okay.
I've been having this pressure in my chest… it comes and goes.

Provider (slight pause, sits down):
I'm really glad you brought that up. Chest pressure is something we should take seriously. Tell me what it feels like.

Patient:
He didn't brush it off; maybe this is important.
It's not constant… but sometimes it worries me.

Provider:
That makes sense. Anyone would feel concerned about that. Let's walk through it carefully, even if we have to be focused.

Patient:
He understands. I don't feel rushed... even though we probably are.
It usually happens when I'm stressed... but once it happened at night too.

Provider (nods):
Okay. That detail matters. I'm going to ask you a few direct questions, so we don't miss anything important.

Patient:
He's moving efficiently... but I feel like he's actually listening.
"Alright."

Provider:
Based on what you're telling me, we should evaluate this further. I don't want to assume it's benign without checking.

Patient:
Good... I was hoping he wouldn't just dismiss it.

Provider (brief pause before concluding):
I know this was a shorter visit, but I want you to feel clear on the plan—and that this concern is being taken seriously.

Patient:
Yes. That's exactly what I needed.

What Made the Difference

The time did not expand. The schedule did not change. But three small, deliberate actions shifted everything:

- A pause before beginning
- A sentence that acknowledged importance
- A moment that reassured presence

The patient did not leave thinking: *That was a short visit.* They left thinking: *I was heard.* And that is the distinction: Patients do not measure care in minutes; they measure it in *attention, intention, and respect.* When those are present, even brief care feels sufficient. When they are absent, even excellent care can feel incomplete.

Chapter 17

Maintaining Humanity in a System That Demands Efficiency

Modern medicine is built on systems designed for movement: schedules to keep, metrics to meet, volumes to sustain. Efficiency is not optional. It is required for access, for throughput, and for the functioning of the entire structure. And yet, within that same system, providers are asked to deliver something that does not naturally conform to efficiency: human connection.

This creates a quiet but constant tension, because humanity in medicine is not expressed through speed. It is expressed through presence, attention, and the willingness to momentarily step out of the purely transactional. The challenge is not that providers forget this. The challenge is that the system rarely pauses long enough to make it easy.

Over time, there is a subtle pressure to adapt. Conversations become streamlined. Language becomes more functional. Interactions begin to center on what is necessary rather than what is meaningful. None of this is inherently wrong. In many ways, it is what allows the system to keep moving. But something important begins to narrow.

The risk is not that care becomes incorrect. The risk is that care becomes *impersonal.* And patients are highly attuned to this distinction. They do not expect unlimited time. They understand, often more than providers realize, that the system is constrained. But what they look for—sometimes without being able to name it—is evidence that within those constraints, they still matter as individuals.

Maintaining humanity, then, is not about resisting efficiency. It is about *embedding humanity within it.* It is a shift in how moments are used, rather than how many moments are available. A provider who maintains humanity in an efficient system does a few things differently:

- They make eye contact before turning to the screen.
- They allow a brief pause before responding.
- They acknowledge emotion even when they cannot fully explore it.
- They signal, in small but unmistakable ways, *"I see you."*

These actions take seconds, but they change the entire tone of the encounter.

A Brief Clinical Contrast

Efficiency without humanity:

Provider:
"What symptoms are you having?"

Patient:
"I've been really anxious… and not sleeping."

Provider:
"Any prior history of anxiety? I'll prescribe something to help with sleep."

(The problem is addressed. The person is not.)

Efficiency with humanity preserved:

Provider (brief pause):
"That sounds exhausting. Not sleeping and feeling anxious can really wear you down."

Patient:
"Yeah… it has been."

Provider:
"I want to help with both the symptoms and what might be driving them. Let's go through this step by step."

The same efficiency. A different experience. The difference is not time. It is intention made visible.

The Deeper Reality

Providers are not asked to carry every emotion, solve every layer, or extend every visit beyond its limits. That would be unsustainable. But they are asked, in each encounter, to make a decision: Will this interaction be purely functional, or will it also be human? That decision is often made in seconds—in tone, in posture and in whether the patient feels like a case—or a person.

Maintaining humanity in a system that demands efficiency is not about doing more; it is about not losing what matters most while doing what is required, because long after the details of a visit fade, patients remember something simpler and more enduring: whether, in a system designed to move quickly, someone chose—if only for a moment—to slow down enough to truly see them.

Part V

Teaching Relationship Skills in Medical Education

Chapter 18	Why Relationship Training Must Start Early	214
Chapter 19	Role-Playing Real Scenarios	216
Chapter 20	Evaluating Communication Skills Objectively	236
Chapter 21	Feedback That Actually Improves Behavior	245
Chapter 22	Integrating Relationship Training into Clinical Rotations	258

Chapter 18

Why Relationship Training Must Start Early

Reframing Priorities in Medical School

The formation of a healthcare provider begins long before the first patient encounter. It begins in the structure of medical education itself, where priorities are quietly established and reinforced over time. Knowledge is measured, tested, and refined with precision. Efficiency is emphasized. Performance is expected. Yet one of the most defining elements of patient care, the ability to build and sustain human connection, is often introduced too late, treated as secondary, or left to develop informally.

This is not an intentional omission. It is a reflection of a system designed to manage complexity, volume, and responsibility. Students are trained to recognize patterns, recall information, and make decisions under pressure. These are essential skills. But without equal attention to relational awareness, something critical is left underdeveloped.

By the time healthcare students reach clinical environments, habits have already formed. They have learned where to focus their attention. They have learned what is evaluated and what is not. If relationship-building is not embedded early, it becomes something they attempt to layer on top of an already demanding cognitive load. Under pressure, it is often the first element to erode.

Early training in relationship-centered care changes this trajectory. It normalizes presence, eye contact, tone, and awareness as fundamental clinical skills rather than optional refinements. It teaches future healthcare providers that how they enter a room, how they acknowledge others, and how they create space for patients to speak are not soft skills, but core competencies.

This shift is not about adding more to an already full curriculum. It is about reframing what is already there. Every standardized patient encounter, every simulation, every bedside interaction becomes an opportunity to reinforce relational habits. Students should not only be evaluated on what they diagnose, but on how they connect, how they listen, and how they are perceived.

When relationship training starts early, it does not compete with clinical excellence. It strengthens it. Patients are more forthcoming. Histories become more accurate. Trust develops more quickly. Care becomes more efficient in a deeper, more meaningful way.

Most importantly, it shapes identity. A healthcare provider who is trained from the beginning to value both knowledge and human connection does not see them as separate. They become integrated. The result is not only better care, but a more grounded, aware, and effective clinician.

If the goal of medical education is to prepare healthcare providers for the realities of practice, then relationship training cannot remain an afterthought. It must be part of the foundation. Because long before patients evaluate what a healthcare provider knows, they experience how that healthcare provider makes them feel. And that experience begins the moment the healthcare provider enters the room.

Chapter 19

Role-Playing Real Scenarios

Teaching Through Experience, Not Theory

There is a limit to what can be learned through instruction alone. Concepts can be explained, frameworks can be outlined, and expectations can be clearly defined. But the moment a provider enters a room with a real patient, variables emerge that no lecture can fully prepare them for. Tone shifts. Emotions surface. Silence carries meaning. It is within these moments that the true complexity of care becomes apparent.

Role-playing real scenarios bridges the gap between knowledge and application. It transforms abstract principles into lived experience. Instead of being told how to communicate, students are placed in situations where they must actively navigate communication. They must decide how to enter the room, how to respond to uncertainty, how to manage multiple people present, and how to recover when something does not go as planned.

This form of training is not about performance. It is about awareness. When students participate in structured role-play, they begin to recognize patterns in themselves. They see where they rush, where they hesitate, where they default to the chart instead of the person. These insights are difficult to access through theory alone. Experience reveals them with clarity.

Equally important is observation and feedback. Watching others navigate the same scenario exposes different approaches to the same moment. Some create immediate ease in the room. Others unintentionally create distance. With guided feedback, students begin to understand not just what they did, but how it was perceived. This distinction is essential. In medicine, intention does not always match impact.

Realistic scenarios should reflect the environments providers will actually encounter. A patient accompanied by family members. A difficult conversation with limited time. A situation where emotions are high and information is incomplete. These are not exceptions in practice. They are the norm.

When role-playing is integrated early and consistently, it reshapes how future providers think about their presence. They begin to see each interaction as dynamic rather than scripted. They learn to adapt without losing structure. They develop the ability to remain composed while still being attentive and responsive.

Over time, these experiences build something that cannot be memorized: instinct. Not instinct in the sense of reaction without thought, but in the sense of familiarity. The room no longer feels unpredictable. It feels navigable.

Teaching through experience ensures that when providers step into real clinical settings, they are not encountering these dynamics for the first time. They have practiced them. They have reflected on them. They have improved within them.

Because in the end, medicine is not only about knowing what to do. It is about knowing how to be in the moment when it matters most.

Role-Playing

These scenarios are not theoretical constructs. They reflect the everyday realities of clinical practice. When rehearsed intentionally, they prepare providers to navigate complexity with clarity, presence, and control.

1. The Delayed Entrance

A provider enters after a long wait. The patient is visibly frustrated, arms crossed, speaking minimally. The task is to acknowledge the delay without becoming defensive and reestablish trust within the first minute.

Provider:
Thank you for your patience. I know the wait was longer than expected.

Patient:
Yeah, it was over an hour.

Provider:
I understand how frustrating that can be. I appreciate you staying.

Patient:
I almost left.

Provider:
I'm glad you didn't. Let's make this time worthwhile.

Patient:
Okay.

Provider:
What brought you in today?

Patient:
I've had this headache for days.

Provider:
That sounds uncomfortable. When did it start?

Patient:
Three days ago.

Provider:
Has anything helped relieve it?

Patient:
Not really.

Provider:
I'm going to ask a few focused questions to understand better.

Patient:
Sure.

Provider:
Any nausea or vision changes?

Patient:
A little nausea.

Provider:
Thank you for sharing that.

Patient:
I just want to feel better.

Provider:
That's our goal today.

Patient:
Okay.

2. The Silent Patient

The patient gives short, minimal answers and avoids eye contact. The challenge is to create psychological safety without forcing conversation.

Provider:
Hi, it's nice to meet you.

Patient:
Hi.

Provider:
What brings you in today?

Patient:
Not sure.

Provider:
That's okay. Take your time.

Patient:
I just don't feel right.

Provider:
Can you tell me more about that feeling?

Patient:
Hard to explain.

Provider:
That's completely fine. We'll figure it out together.

Patient:
Okay.

Provider:
When did this start?

Patient:
A few weeks ago.

Provider:
Any changes in sleep or appetite?

Patient:
Yeah, both.

Provider:
Thank you for sharing that.

Patient:
I don't talk about this much.

Provider:
You're in a safe place to do so.

Patient:
That helps.

Provider:
We'll go step by step.

Patient:
Alright.

3. The Over-Talking Family Member

A parent or partner answers every question before the patient can speak. The provider must respectfully redirect focus back to the patient while maintaining inclusion.

Provider:
What brings you in today?

Patient:
I've been—

Patient's Mother:
She's been coughing nonstop!

Provider:
I appreciate that. Let me hear from her first.

Patient:
It started last week.

Provider:
Thank you. Go ahead.

Patient:
It's worse at night.

Patient's Mother:
And she barely sleeps!

Provider:
That's helpful, thank you. I'll come back to you shortly.

Patient:
Yeah, nights are tough.

Provider:
Any fever?

Patient:
A little.

Provider:
Thank you.

Patient's Mother:
I was worried it's serious.

Provider:
Your concern is important.

Patient:
I just want it checked.

Provider:
That's exactly what we'll do.

Patient:
Okay.

Provider:
We'll address both of your concerns.

4. The Anxious First-Time Patient

A young patient appears overwhelmed and nervous. The provider must slow the pace, normalize the experience, and reduce anxiety.

Provider:
Hi, I'm glad you came in today.

Patient:
I'm really nervous.

Provider:
That's completely normal.

Patient:
I don't like doctors.

Provider:
Many people feel that way.

Patient:
Okay.

Provider:
We'll go at your pace.

Patient:
That helps.

Provider:
What's been bothering you?

Patient:
My chest feels tight.

Provider:
When did that start?

Patient:
Yesterday.

Provider:
We'll check everything carefully.

Patient:
Okay.

Provider:
You're in control here.

Patient:
Thank you.

Provider:
We'll take this step by step.

Patient:
I appreciate that.

Provider:
You're doing great.

Patient:
Thanks.

5. The Distrustful Patient

The patient questions recommendations and references negative past experiences with healthcare. The goal is to respond without defensiveness and build credibility.

Provider:
What brings you in today?

Patient:
Doctors never help me.

Provider:
I'm sorry you've had that experience.

Patient:
It's always the same.

Provider:
I'd like to understand your concerns.

Patient:
I don't trust this process.

Provider:
That's fair to say.

Patient:
So what's different now?

Provider:
I'll listen carefully and explain clearly.

Patient:
We'll see.

Provider:
What symptoms are you having?

Patient:
Constant fatigue.

Provider:
How long has this been going on?

Patient:
Months.

Provider:
Let's work through it together.

Patient:
Alright.

Provider:
You deserve clarity.

Patient:
I hope so.

Provider:
That's what we'll aim for.

6. The Emotional Disclosure

Mid-visit, the patient becomes tearful and shares a personal struggle unrelated to the chief complaint. The provider must balance empathy with maintaining clinical structure.

Provider:
What brings you in today?

Patient:
I've been feeling sick...

Provider:
Tell me more.

Patient:
(tearful) I've been really stressed.

Provider:
Take your time.

Patient:
Everything feels overwhelming.

Provider:
That sounds very difficult.

Patient:
I didn't expect to cry.

Provider:
It's okay to feel this way.

Patient:
Thank you.

Provider:
We can address both your physical and emotional concerns.

Patient:
That would help.

Provider:
When did this start?

Patient:
A few weeks ago.

Provider:
You're not alone in this.

Patient:
I needed to hear that.

Provider:
We'll take this one step at a time.

Patient:
Okay.

Provider:
I'm here with you.

Patient:
Thank you.

7. The Time-Pressured Visit

The provider is running behind, but the patient presents multiple concerns. The task is to prioritize without making the patient feel dismissed.

Provider:
I want to respect your time today. What's most important to address?

Patient:
I have a few things.

Provider:
Let's prioritize together.

Patient:
My back pain first.

Provider:
Okay, let's start there.

Patient:
It's been bad lately.

Provider:
When did it worsen?

Patient:
Last week.

Provider:
Any injuries?

Patient:
No.

Provider:
We'll focus on that first.

Patient:
I also have headaches.

Provider:
Let's schedule a follow-up for that.

Patient:
That works.

Provider:
I want to give each issue proper attention.

Patient:
I appreciate that.

Provider:
Let's address your back thoroughly today.

Patient:
Okay.

Provider:
We'll make a plan.

8. The Language Barrier

The patient has limited English proficiency, with a family member attempting to translate. The provider must manage clarity, accuracy, and patient-centered communication.

Provider:
Hello, I'm glad you're here.

Patient:
(speaks limited English)

Translator (Family):
She has stomach pain.

Provider:
Thank you. I'd like to speak directly to her as well.

Patient:
(nods)

Provider:
Can you point to where it hurts?

Patient:
(points)

Provider:
Thank you.

Translator:
It started yesterday.

Provider:
I appreciate your help.

Provider:
(to patient) Pain now?

Patient:
Yes.

Provider:
We'll take care of this.

Translator:
She is worried.

Provider:
That's understandable.

Provider:
We'll explain each step.

Patient:
Thank you.

Provider:
You're in good hands.

Patient:
Okay.

9. The Technology Distraction

The provider is tempted to focus on the computer while documenting. The exercise emphasizes maintaining presence while integrating technology.

Provider:
What brings you in today?

Patient:
I've been dizzy.

Provider:
(turns away from screen) Tell me more.

Patient:
It happens when I stand up.

Provider:
How often?

Patient:
Every day.

Provider:
I'm listening.

Patient:
It's getting worse.

Provider:
Thank you for explaining.

Provider:
I'll take notes after we talk.

Patient:
That feels better.

Provider:
When did it begin?

Patient:
A week ago.

Provider:
Any other symptoms?

Patient:
No.

Provider:
We'll evaluate this carefully.

Patient:
Okay.

Provider:
You have my full attention.

Patient:
I appreciate that.

10. The Non-Adherent Patient

The patient has not followed previous recommendations. The provider must explore reasons without judgment and encourage re-engagement.

Provider:
How have things been since your last visit?

Patient:
I didn't follow the plan.

Provider:
Thank you for being honest.

Patient:
It was hard.

Provider:
Tell me what got in the way.

Patient:
I forgot and got busy.

Provider:
That happens.

Patient:
I feel bad about it.

Provider:
No judgment here.

Patient:
Okay.

Provider:
Let's adjust the plan.

Patient:
That would help.

Provider:
What feels realistic for you?

Patient:
Something simpler.

Provider:
We can do that.

Patient:
Thank you.

Provider:
We'll build something sustainable.

Patient:
I appreciate it.

11. The Dominant Personality

A confident, assertive patient attempts to control the direction of the visit. The provider must maintain structure without creating conflict.

Provider:
What brings you in today?

Patient:
I already know what I need.

Provider:
I'm happy to hear your thoughts.

Patient:
I need a specific medication.

Provider:
Let's review your symptoms first.

Patient:
I've done my research.

Provider:
That's valuable.

Patient:
So just prescribe it.

Provider:
My role is to ensure it's appropriate.

Patient:
Fine.

Provider:
Tell me your symptoms.

Patient:
Persistent cough.

Provider:
Let's examine that carefully.

Patient:
Okay.

Provider:
We'll decide together.

Patient:
That's fair.

Provider:
I want the best outcome for you.

Patient:
Alright.

12. The Sensitive Topic

The discussion involves a stigmatized issue, such as substance use or sexual health. The provider must approach with neutrality and professionalism.

Provider:
I'd like to discuss something personal.

Patient:
Okay.

Provider:
Everything here is confidential.

Patient:
That helps.

Provider:
Have you used any substances recently?

Patient:
Yes.

Provider:
Thank you for your honesty.

Patient:
I was nervous to say it.

Provider:
No judgment here.

Patient:
Okay.

Provider:
We're focused on your health.

Patient:
I understand.

Provider:
How often?

Patient:
Occasionally.

Provider:
We'll discuss safe next steps.

Patient:
Thank you.

Provider:
You did the right thing sharing.

Patient:
I feel relieved.

13. The Multi-Person Room

The patient is accompanied by multiple family members with differing opinions. The provider must manage the room while keeping the patient central.

Provider:
Thank you all for being here.

Patient:
It's helpful to have them.

Family Member 1:
We're concerned.

Family Member 2:
Very concerned.

Provider:
I understand.

Provider:
Let's hear from the patient first.

Patient:
I've been feeling weak.

Provider:
Thank you.

Family Member 1:
She barely eats.

Provider:
I'll come back to that.

Provider (to patient):
Tell me more.

Patient:
I have no appetite.

Provider:
That's important.

Family Member 2:
We've noticed weight loss.

Provider:
Thank you.

Provider:
I'll address all concerns.

Patient:
Okay.

Provider:
We'll work as a team.

14. The Unexpected Anger

The patient expresses frustration or raises their voice about prior care. The provider must de-escalate while maintaining professionalism.

Provider:
What brings you in today?

Patient:
I'm frustrated with this system.

Provider:
I hear that.

Patient:
No one listens.

Provider:
I'm here to listen now.

Patient:
It's been awful.

Provider:
That sounds very difficult.

Patient:
I'm tired of it.

Provider:
Let's focus on what we can improve today.

Patient:
Okay.

Provider:
Tell me what's been happening.

Patient:
Constant pain.

Provider:
I want to understand fully.

Patient:
Thank you.

Provider:
We'll work through this together.

Patient:
I hope so.

Provider:
That's our goal.

15. The Closing Moment

The visit is ending, but the patient hesitates and says, "One more thing…" The provider must decide how to handle additional concerns without rushing or dismissing.

Provider:
We've covered a lot today.

Patient:
Yes.

Provider:
Any final questions?

Patient:
Actually… one more thing.

Provider:
I'm glad you mentioned it.

Patient:
I've had trouble sleeping.

Provider:
Tell me more.

Patient:
It's been weeks.

Provider:
Thank you for bringing it up.

Patient:
I wasn't sure.

Provider:
This is important.

Patient:
Okay.

Provider:
Let's address it briefly now.

Patient:
Thank you.

Provider:
We can also follow up if needed.

Patient:
That works.

Provider:
I'm glad you spoke up.

Patient:
Me too.

Chapter 20

Evaluating Communication Skills Objectively

What Should Be Measured—And How

Communication in healthcare has long been described as essential, yet it is rarely measured with the same precision as clinical knowledge. What is not measured consistently becomes variable, and what is variable becomes unreliable. If communication is to be treated as a core clinical skill, it must be evaluated with clarity, structure, and objectivity.

The challenge is not recognizing its importance. The challenge is defining it in a way that can be observed, assessed, and improved without reducing it to something artificial or performative. Communication is not a single behavior. It is a sequence of observable actions that occur within a defined timeframe, particularly in the opening, middle, and closing of an encounter.

Example: Measuring Initial Presence in Real Time

The first domain to measure is **initial presence.** This includes how the provider enters the room, whether they pause, establish eye contact, and acknowledge all individuals present. These behaviors occur within seconds, yet they set the tone for the entire interaction. They are visible, repeatable, and measurable.

The provider approaches the exam room door, pauses briefly, and takes a breath before entering. This moment is not visible to the patient, but it prepares the provider to be fully present.

The provider enters the room without looking at the chart or computer. Their posture is upright, unhurried, and oriented toward the people in the room.

Within the first two seconds, the provider lifts their gaze and makes direct eye contact with the patient.

Provider:
Good morning.

The tone is calm, clear, and unhurried. The provider maintains eye contact for a moment, allowing the greeting to land before speaking again.

Provider:
Hi, I'm Dr. Harris. It's nice to meet you.

The provider then shifts their gaze naturally to the others in the room, without losing connection to the patient.

Provider:
And you are?

Each individual is acknowledged with a brief nod and eye contact as they introduce themselves.

Provider:
Thank you for being here.

The provider then returns their primary focus to the patient. Before proceeding further, the provider establishes clarity and respect for boundaries.

Provider:
Are you comfortable discussing everything with them in the room?

The patient responds affirmatively. The provider nods, maintaining a composed and attentive posture. At no point during this sequence does the provider look down at the chart, adjust equipment, or turn away from the people in the room. The entire interaction takes less than ten seconds.

What has been demonstrated is measurable:

- Eye contact established within two seconds.
- All individuals acknowledged within five seconds.
- Roles identified within seven seconds.
- Consent confirmed before clinical discussion begins.

The result is not simply a polite introduction. It is a structured, repeatable sequence that signals awareness, respect, and control from the very first moment of the encounter.

Example:Measuring Patient-Centered Engagement in Real Time

The second domain is **patient-centered engagement.** This evaluates whether the provider allows the patient to speak without interruption, demonstrates active listening, and responds in a way that reflects understanding. It is not enough to ask questions. The quality of listening and the appropriateness of responses must be assessed.

The provider has completed the initial orientation and now transitions fully into the patient's narrative without interruption or redirection.

Provider:
Tell me what's been going on.

The question is open-ended, allowing the patient to define the starting point rather than being guided prematurely.

Patient:
I've been having this pressure in my chest for a few days, and it's been worrying me.

The provider maintains steady eye contact, nodding subtly, without typing or looking away. There is no interruption. A brief pause follows as the patient continues.

Patient:
It started after I was walking, and now I notice it even when I'm resting.

The provider allows the patient to complete their thought fully. Only after the patient finishes does the provider respond.

Provider:
You've been feeling chest pressure for a few days, and it started with activity but now happens even at rest. That sounds concerning.

This response reflects *active listening*. It demonstrates that the provider has not only heard the words, but understood their significance. The provider's tone is measured and validating, not alarmist or dismissive.

Patient:
Yes, exactly.

The provider continues to build on the patient's narrative rather than redirecting abruptly.

Provider:
What worried you most when you noticed this?

This question deepens the patient's perspective rather than narrowing it too quickly.

Patient:
I was afraid it might be something serious with my heart.

The provider acknowledges the emotional component explicitly.

Provider:
That's a very understandable concern.

Again, there is no interruption, no immediate pivot to testing or diagnosis. The provider allows space before proceeding. Only after the patient feels heard does the provider begin more structured questioning.

What has been demonstrated is measurable:

- The patient was allowed to speak without interruption for the initial narrative.
- The provider maintained a visual and physical presence throughout.
- The provider reflected back key elements accurately.
- The provider acknowledged both the clinical concern and the emotional context.

This is not passive listening. It is deliberate, structured engagement that ensures the patient's voice is not only heard, but understood and integrated into care.

Example: Measuring Relational Awareness in Real Time

The third domain is **relational awareness**. This includes how the provider manages others in the room, confirms consent for shared discussion, and balances attention without losing focus on the patient. These are subtle but critical indicators of professionalism and control.

The provider has completed the initial greeting and is now aware that multiple people are present in the room. The patient is accompanied by her mother and partner.

Provider:
Before we go further, I just want to confirm, are you comfortable discussing everything with them here in the room?

The provider directs this question clearly to the patient, maintaining eye contact and a neutral, respectful tone.

Patient:
Yes, that's okay.

The provider nods, acknowledging the patient's authority in the decision.

Provider:
Thank you.

The provider subtly shifts posture to include the others in the room without redirecting control away from the patient.

Provider:
I appreciate you both being here to support her.

Brief eye contact is made with each accompanying person, signaling inclusion without shifting the center of attention.

The provider then returns primary focus to the patient.

Provider:
Can you tell me what's been going on?

The patient begins speaking but is interrupted by their mother.

Mother:
She's been having pain for days—

The provider gently raises a hand slightly and redirects with calm clarity.

Provider:
I'm going to start with her, and then I'll make sure to hear from you as well.

The tone remains respectful, not corrective.

The patient continues.

Patient:
It started earlier this week.

The provider listens attentively, maintaining primary eye contact with the patient while occasionally acknowledging others with brief glances.

After the patient finishes her initial explanation, the provider reopens the space to others.

Provider:
Is there anything either of you have noticed that you think would be helpful for me to know?

The mother responds.

Mother:
She hasn't been sleeping well.

The provider nods.

Provider:
That's helpful, thank you.

The provider returns focus to the patient again, maintaining a clear structure.

What has been demonstrated is measurable:

- Consent for the shared discussion was explicitly confirmed before proceeding.
- The patient remained the central focus throughout the interaction.
- Accompanying individuals were acknowledged and respectfully included.
- Interruptions were redirected without creating tension or dismissal.
- Attention was balanced without losing control of the encounter.

This is relational awareness in practice. It reflects not only politeness, but deliberate management of the interpersonal dynamics within the room.

Example: Measuring Clarity of Communication in Real Time

The fourth domain is **clarity of communication.** Information should be conveyed in a way that is understandable, structured, and appropriately paced. Medical language must be translated without condescension. The patient should leave with a clear understanding of their condition and next steps.

The provider has gathered the history and completed the examination. The patient is waiting for an explanation. The provider pauses briefly, making direct eye contact before speaking, ensuring the patient is ready to receive information.

Provider:
I'm going to walk you through what I think is happening, and then we'll talk about what we do next.

The statement sets structure and prepares the patient.

Patient:
Okay.

Provider:
The pressure you're feeling in your chest does not appear to be coming from your heart based on what we've seen so far.

The provider avoids complex terminology and begins with a clear, direct conclusion. The patient visibly relaxes.

Provider:
Instead, it's more consistent with inflammation of the muscles between your ribs. It can feel alarming, but it's not dangerous.

The provider translates the concept into plain language and immediately addresses emotional concern.

Patient:
So it's not my heart?

Provider:
Correct. Based on your exam and symptoms, there's no sign of a heart problem right now.

The provider confirms understanding without dismissing the patient's fear. The provider continues in a structured sequence.

Provider:
Here's what we're going to do next. First, I'll recommend an anti-inflammatory medication to reduce the discomfort. Second, I want you to avoid heavy lifting for a few days. Third, if anything changes, like worsening pain or new symptoms, you should contact us right away.

The steps are clearly numbered, paced, and easy to follow. The provider pauses.

Provider:
Can you tell me, in your own words, what the plan is?

This checks understanding without testing or intimidating the patient.

Patient:
It's not my heart, it's muscle-related. I take the medication, rest, and call if it gets worse.

Provider:
Exactly.

The provider nods, reinforcing clarity.

Provider:
Do you have any questions or anything that doesn't feel clear?

Patient:
No, that makes sense.

What has been demonstrated is measurable:

- Information was delivered in clear, non-technical language.
- The explanation followed a logical and structured sequence.
- Emotional concerns were addressed alongside clinical facts.

- The patient was asked to repeat the plan to confirm understanding.
- The pace allowed time for processing and questions.

This is clarity of communication. It ensures that understanding is not assume, but confirmed, and that the patient leaves not only informed but confident in what comes next.

Example: Measuring Closure and Alignment in Real Time

The fifth domain is **closure and alignment.** The provider should confirm understanding, invite final questions, and ensure that the patient feels heard and supported before the encounter ends. The closing moments are as important as the opening, yet often rushed or overlooked.

The clinical discussion has concluded, and the provider transitions deliberately into the closing phase rather than ending abruptly. The provider maintains eye contact and slightly leans forward, signaling continued presence.

Provider:
Before we finish, I want to make sure we're aligned on everything we discussed.

The tone is calm and unhurried.

Patient:
Okay.

Provider:
Can you tell me what your understanding is of what's going on and what the plan is?

The question is open and respectful, allowing the patient to summarize without pressure.

Patient:
It's muscle-related, not my heart. I'll take the medication, rest, and call if anything changes.

The provider nods, reinforcing accuracy.

Provider:
That's exactly right.

A brief pause follows, allowing space for additional thoughts.

Provider:
What questions do you still have?

The wording assumes there may be questions, making it easier for the patient to speak.

Patient:
No, I think that covered it.

The provider does not rush to exit.

Provider:
Is there anything we didn't talk about that you were hoping to address today?

This creates a final opportunity for overlooked concerns.

Patient:
No, I feel good about it.

The provider acknowledges the patient's emotional state as well as the clinical plan.

Provider:
I'm glad. You did the right thing coming in.

The provider offers reassurance without exaggeration.

Provider:
If anything changes or you feel uncertain, don't hesitate to reach out. We're here for you.

The statement reinforces ongoing support. The provider maintains eye contact for a final moment before standing.

Provider:
Take care of yourself, and we'll follow up as planned.

The exit is calm, intentional, and complete.

What has been demonstrated is measurable:

- The provider confirmed understanding through patient explanation.
- Final questions were invited in an open, non-restrictive way.
- Additional concerns were proactively explored.
- Emotional reassurance was provided appropriately.
- The encounter ended with clear support and next steps.

This is closure and alignment. It ensures that the patient does not leave with uncertainty, but with clarity, confidence, and a sense of being fully cared for.

To evaluate these domains objectively, structured tools must be used. Standardized checklists, direct observation, and recorded encounters can provide measurable data. Each domain can be broken down into specific behaviors: Did the provider make eye contact within the first five seconds? Did they interrupt the patient? Did they confirm understanding before closing?

Importantly, evaluation must include both **what was done** and **how it was perceived**. A technically correct interaction may still feel distant or rushed. Incorporating patient feedback adds a necessary dimension that purely observational metrics cannot capture.

Consistency in evaluation creates consistency in performance. When students and providers know that communication is being assessed with the same rigor as diagnosis, it becomes integrated into their practice rather than treated as optional.

Objective evaluation does not diminish the human element of communication. It protects it. It ensures that the qualities patients value most — presence, respect, clarity — are not left to chance, but are developed, reinforced, and sustained over time, because in clinical practice, how something is said is not separate from what is said. It is part of the care itself.

Chapter 21

Feedback That Actually Improves Behavior

Feedback is one of the most frequently given and least effectively used tools in medical training. It is often delivered with good intention, yet without structure, specificity, or timing, it fails to produce meaningful change. When feedback is vague, delayed, or overly generalized, it becomes something learners acknowledge but do not integrate. For feedback to improve behavior, it must be **observable, specific, and immediately actionable**.

Example: Feedback to Behavior, Not Personality

The first principle is **anchoring feedback to behavior, not personality.** Saying "you were disengaged" is subjective and difficult to act on. Saying "you looked at the computer for the first 20 seconds without making eye contact" is precise, measurable, and correctable. The learner knows exactly what occurred and what can be changed.

A medical student has just completed a patient encounter while the attending healthcare provider observed quietly from the corner of the room. After stepping out of the room and walking down the hallway, they pause.

Attending Healthcare Provider:
Before I share anything, how do you think that went?

Medical Student:
I think it was okay. I got the history.

Attending Healthcare Provider:
You did gather the key information.

A brief pause follows.

Attending Healthcare Provider:
I want to point out one specific moment I observed.

The framing is neutral and focused.

Medical Student:
Okay.

Attending Healthcare Provider:
When you entered the room, you spent about the first 20 seconds looking at the computer and reviewing the chart before making eye contact with the patient.

The feedback is precise, time-bound, and observable.

Medical Student:
Oh… I didn't realize that.

Attending Healthcare Provider:
During that time, the patient was watching you and didn't speak.

The attending links behavior to impact.

Medical Student:
I see.

Attending Healthcare Provider:
Instead of starting with the computer, try this:
pause, look at the patient first, and say, 'Hi, I'm ___, it's good to meet you,' before turning to the chart.

The replacement behavior is clear and actionable.

Medical Student:
That makes sense.

Attending Healthcare Provider:
It's a small shift, but it changes how the patient experiences the entire visit.

Medical Student:
I can do that.

Attending Healthcare Provider:
Let's try it that way on the next patient.

What has been demonstrated is measurable:

- The feedback focused on a specific, observable behavior.
- The timing and duration of the behavior were clearly identified.
- The impact on the patient was explained.
- A direct alternative behavior was provided.
- The learner understood exactly what to change and how to change it.

This is feedback that can be applied immediately, repeated consistently, and improved upon with each encounter.

Example: Timing of Feedback in Real Time

The second principle is **timing**. Feedback should occur as close to the observed behavior as possible. When delivered immediately after an encounter, the details are still clear, and the learner can connect the feedback directly to their actions. Delayed feedback loses impact and becomes abstract.

A resident completes a patient encounter involving a difficult conversation. As soon as they step out of the room, the attending healthcare provider walks with them a few steps down the hallway and pauses.

Attending Healthcare Provider:
Let's take a minute while that's still fresh.

The timing is immediate, anchored to the just-completed interaction.

Resident:
Okay.

Attending Healthcare Provider:
How do you think that conversation went?

Resident:
I think it was okay, but I felt a bit rushed.

Attending Healthcare Provider:
You handled the explanation clearly.

A brief pause follows.

Attending Healthcare Provider:
There's one moment I want to focus on while it's still clear.

Resident:
Sure.

Attending Healthcare Provider:
When the patient started asking about risks, you shifted quickly to the next topic without

addressing her concern directly.

The feedback references a specific, recent moment.

Resident:
Yeah, I remember that.

Attending Healthcare Provider:
Right then, she paused and looked uncertain.

The attending connects the behavior to what just occurred.

Resident:
I noticed that too.

Attending Healthcare Provider:
In that moment, a simple response like, 'That's an important question, let's go through that together,' would have helped her feel heard.

Resident:
That makes sense.

Attending Healthcare Provider:
Because we're talking about it immediately, you can probably picture that exact moment.

Resident:
I can.

Attending Healthcare Provider:
That's why timing matters. You can adjust it on your very next patient.

Resident:
I will.

Attending Healthcare Provider:
Let's try that approach right away.

What has been demonstrated is measurable:

- Feedback was delivered immediately after the encounter.
- The specific moment was still clear in the learner's mind.
- The learner was able to recall the exact interaction without prompting.
- The connection between behavior and impact was immediate and concrete.
- A correction can be applied in the very next clinical interaction.

This is effective timing. It transforms feedback from something remembered vaguely into something that can be visualized, understood, and immediately improved.

Example: Focused Feedback on One Key Behavior

The third principle is **focus.** Effective feedback targets one or two key behaviors rather than overwhelming the learner with multiple corrections. Depth is more valuable than breadth. When too many points are raised at once, none are fully integrated.

A medical student completes a patient encounter that included several areas for improvement. The attending healthcare provider steps aside with the student immediately afterward.

Attending Healthcare Provider:
Before I give feedback, how do you think that went?

Medical Student:
I think I did okay, but I might have missed some things.

Attending Healthcare Provider:
You gathered a thorough history, which was good.

A brief pause follows, signaling a shift to focused feedback.

Attending Healthcare Provider:
I'm going to focus on one thing that will make the biggest difference right now.

The scope is intentionally narrowed.

Medical Student:
Okay.

Attending Healthcare Provider:
During the first minute, you interrupted the patient twice while they were describing their symptoms.

The feedback is specific and limited to a single behavior.

Medical Student:
I didn't realize I did that.

Attending Healthcare provider:
It's common, especially when you're trying to guide the conversation.

The tone remains supportive.

Attending Healthcare Provider:
When you interrupted, the patient stopped mid-sentence and didn't return to that detail.

The impact is clearly linked.

Medical Student:
I see.

Attending Healthcare provider:
For now, I want you to focus on one adjustment:
let the patient speak for at least 20 to 30 seconds without interruption at the start.

The correction is simple and actionable.

Medical Student:
I can do that.

Attending Healthcare provider:
We'll work on other areas later, but this one change will improve your entire interaction.

Medical Student:
That helps to focus.

Attending Healthcare provider:
Try it on your next patient.

What has been demonstrated is measurable:

- Only one key behavior was addressed.
- The feedback was specific and clearly defined.
- The learner was not overwhelmed with multiple corrections.
- A single, actionable adjustment was provided.
- The likelihood of immediate application and improvement is high.

This is focused feedback. It prioritizes depth over breadth, allowing meaningful change to occur one behavior at a time.

Example: Demonstration and Replacement in Feedback

The fourth principle is **demonstration and replacement.** It is not enough to point out what was ineffective. The learner must be shown what to do instead. This can be done through modeling, role-play, or simple phrasing. For example, replacing "What's wrong?" with "Tell me what's been going on" changes the entire tone of the interaction.

A resident completes a patient encounter while the attending observes. Afterward, they step aside to discuss.

Attending Healthcare Provider:
How do you think that went?

Resident:
I think it was fine, but the patient seemed a little closed off.

Attending Healthcare Provider:
You gathered the necessary information, but I want to focus on how you opened the visit.

Resident:
Okay.

Attending Healthcare Provider:
You started by asking, "What's wrong?"

The feedback identifies the exact behavior.

Resident:
Yes.

Attending Healthcare Provider:
That question can sometimes feel abrupt or limiting to patients.

The attending briefly explains the impact.

Resident:
I didn't think about that.

Attending Healthcare Provider:
Let me show you a simple alternative.

The attending shifts into demonstration.

Attending Healthcare Provider (modeling):
Instead of "What's wrong?" try, "Tell me what's been going on."

The tone is calm, open, and inviting.

Resident:
That does sound different.

Attending Healthcare Provider:
It gives the patient more space and signals that you're ready to listen.

Resident:
I see that.

Attending Healthcare Provider:
Let's role-play it for a moment.

Resident:
Okay.

The attending healthcare provider takes on the role of the patient, sitting quietly.

Resident:
Tell me what's been going on.

Attending Healthcare Provider:
That's it. Notice how that feels more open?

Resident:
Yes, it does.

Attending Healthcare Provider:
Use that phrasing on your next patient.

Resident:
I will.

What has been demonstrated is measurable:

- The ineffective behavior was clearly identified.
- A specific replacement phrase was provided.
- The attending modeled the improved behavior.
- The learner practiced the new approach immediately.
- The change is simple, repeatable, and applicable in the next encounter.

This is demonstration and replacement. It transforms feedback from critique into a practical tool for immediate improvement.

Example: Self-Reflection Before Correction

The fifth principle is **self-reflection before correction**. Asking the learner, "How do you think that went?" encourages awareness and ownership. Often, learners recognize their own gaps when given space to reflect. Feedback then becomes a refinement rather than a correction imposed from outside.

A medical student finishes a patient encounter while the attending healthcare provider observes quietly. They step into the hallway immediately afterward. The attending does not begin with correction.

Attending Healthcare Provider:
How do you think that went?

The question is open, neutral, and non-judgmental.

Medical Student:
I think it was okay… but I felt like I was rushing.

The learner begins identifying their own perception.

Attending Healthcare Provider:
What made it feel rushed to you?

The attending deepens reflection rather than redirecting.

Medical Student:
I didn't give the patient much time to talk at the beginning.

Attending Healthcare provider:
What did you notice when that happened?

Medical Student:
They gave shorter answers after that.

The learner connects behavior to impact independently.

Attending Healthcare Provider:
That's an important observation.

A brief pause allows the insight to settle.

Medical Student:
I think I interrupted too early.

Attending Healthcare Provider:
I agree with that.

Now the attending aligns with the learner's self-identified gap.

Attending Healthcare provider:
What might you try differently next time?

The learner is guided toward solution-building.

Medical Student:
Let them speak longer before I jump in.

Attending Healthcare provider:
That would be a strong adjustment.

The feedback now reinforces, rather than imposes.

Attending Healthcare provider:
If you allow even 20 to 30 seconds without interruption, you'll likely get more complete information.

Medical Student:
That makes sense.

Attending Healthcare provider:
Let's try that on your next patient.

What has been demonstrated is measurable:

- The learner was prompted to self-assess before receiving feedback.
- The attending guided reflection through focused questions.
- The learner independently identified the key issue.
- Correction emerged as reinforcement rather than external critique.
- Ownership of improvement remained with the learner.

This is self-reflection before correction. It transforms feedback into a collaborative process, where awareness leads the way and change becomes internally driven.

Example: Linking Behavior to Impact

The sixth principle is **linking behavior to impact.** Learners are more likely to change when they understand not just what they did, but how it was perceived. For example, "When you interrupted after three seconds, the patient stopped sharing important details" connects action to consequence.

A resident completes a patient encounter while the attending healthcare provider observes. After stepping out of the room, they pause to discuss.

Attending Healthcare Provider:
How do you think that went?

Resident:
I think it was okay. I got most of the information.

Attending Healthcare Provider:
You did gather several important points.

A brief pause follows.

Attending Healthcare Provider:
I want to focus on one specific moment.

Resident:
Okay.

Attending Healthcare Provider:
At the beginning of the visit, the patient started describing her symptoms, and after about three seconds, you interrupted to ask a more specific question.

The behavior is clearly identified and time bound.

Resident:
I didn't realize it was that quick.

Attending Healthcare Provider:
Right after that interruption, she stopped expanding on her symptoms and began giving shorter, more limited answers.

The attending connects the behavior directly to its impact.

Resident:
Now that you say that, I noticed she became quieter.

Attending Healthcare Provider:
Exactly. When patients are interrupted early, they often assume they should limit what they share.

The consequence is explained in practical terms.

Resident:
That makes sense.

Attending Healthcare Provider:
If you allow the patient to speak uninterrupted for even 20 to 30 seconds, you'll often get more complete and useful information.

Resident:
I can see how that would help.

Attending Healthcare Provider:
So the adjustment isn't just about waiting longer. It's about what that extra time allows the patient to give you.

Resident:
That's a different way to think about it.

Attending Healthcare Provider:
Try that on your next encounter and notice how the patient responds.

What has been demonstrated is measurable:

- A specific behavior was identified with clear timing.
- The direct impact on the patient's behavior was explained.
- The learner recognized the change in patient response.
- The connection between action and consequence was made explicit.
- The adjustment is tied to improved clinical outcomes.

This is linking behavior to impact. It moves feedback beyond correction and into understanding, where change becomes both logical and meaningful.

Example: Repetition and Reinforcement in Feedback

The final principle is **repetition and reinforcement.** Behavior does not change with a single comment. It changes through consistent feedback, practice, and reinforcement over time. What is repeated becomes habit.

A medical student has been working on improving how they open patient encounters, specifically allowing the patient to speak without interruption. This is not their first feedback session on this behavior. After a morning clinic session, the attending healthcare provider meets briefly with the student.

Attending Healthcare Provider:
Let's revisit the opening of your encounters today.

The focus is consistent with prior feedback.

Medical Student:
I've been trying to let the patient talk longer.

Attending Healthcare Provider:
I noticed that.

A brief pause reinforces progress.

Attending Healthcare Provider:
On your first patient, you allowed about 10 seconds before speaking.

Medical Student:
That's better than before.

Attending Healthcare Provider:
It is. Last time, it was closer to three seconds.

The attending references prior performance, showing continuity.

Medical Student:
I'm trying to be more aware.

Attending Healthcare Provider:
On your second patient, you extended that to nearly 20 seconds.

Medical Student:
I did feel like I got more information.

Attending Healthcare Provider:
You did. The patient shared more detail without prompting.

The improvement is linked to outcome.

Medical Student:
That was noticeable.

Attending Healthcare Provider:
This is exactly how habits form. Repetition with small adjustments.

The principle is made explicit.

Medical Student:
So I should keep aiming for that?

Attending Healthcare Provider:
Yes. Let's keep reinforcing that 20 to 30 second window.

Medical Student:
Okay.

Attending Healthcare Provider:
We'll check it again tomorrow.

The feedback is ongoing, not one-time.

Medical Student:
That helps me stay focused.

Attending Healthcare Provider:
You're building consistency. That's what turns effort into habit.

What has been demonstrated is measurable:

- The same behavior was revisited across multiple encounters.
- Progress was tracked and compared over time.
- Improvement was reinforced with specific observations.
- The learner practiced repeatedly with incremental gains.
- Feedback was positioned as an ongoing process, not a single event.

This is repetition and reinforcement. It ensures that change is not temporary, but sustained, becoming a natural and reliable part of clinical practice.

When feedback is delivered with this level of clarity and intention, it shifts from evaluation to development. It becomes something learners seek rather than avoid, because in clinical practice, improvement does not come from knowing what is right; it comes from repeatedly seeing, understanding, and adjusting what is actually done.

Chapter 22

Integrating Relationship Training into Clinical Rotations

Clinical rotations are where medical training becomes real. It is the point at which knowledge is no longer theoretical, but applied in dynamic, unpredictable environments. Students move from classrooms into patient rooms, from structured learning into lived experience. It is here, more than anywhere else, that habits are formed.

Yet within this critical phase, relationship training is often left unstructured. Students are expected to "pick it up" by observation, to model what they see, and to adapt intuitively. This approach creates inconsistency. Some learners develop strong relational skills. Others, equally capable academically, struggle without ever receiving clear guidance.

Integration requires intention.

Relationship training must be embedded into the daily workflow of clinical rotations, not added as a separate or optional component. It should be present in every patient encounter, every observation, and every feedback session. The goal is not to create additional tasks, but to redefine what is already being done.

Example: Making Relationship Behaviors Visible in Real Time

The first step is **making relationship behaviors visible.** Preceptors should explicitly name what they are doing in real time. A simple statement such as, "I'm going to pause and make eye contact before I speak," transforms an invisible habit into a teachable moment. When learners can see and understand the structure behind the behavior, they can begin to replicate it.

Preceptor:
Before we go into the room, I want you to watch something specific.

Medical Student:
Okay.

Preceptor:
When I enter, I'm going to pause, look up, and make eye contact before I say anything.

Medical Student:
Got it.

(The preceptor gently knocks and enters the room.)

Preceptor (pauses, looks directly at patient):
Good morning.

Patient:
Good morning.

Preceptor:
Hi, I'm Dr. Harris. It's nice to meet you.

(The preceptor briefly acknowledges the family member with eye contact.)

Preceptor:
And you are?

Family Member:
I'm her mother.

Preceptor:
Thank you for being here.

(The preceptor turns slightly back toward the patient.)

Preceptor:
Are you comfortable discussing everything with her in the room?

Patient:
Yes.

(The encounter continues briefly, then transitions out of the room.)

Preceptor:
What did you notice when I walked in?

Medical Student:
You didn't look at the chart first. You looked at the patient.

Preceptor:
Exactly. I paused and made eye contact before speaking.

Medical Student:
It felt more personal.

Preceptor:
That pause is intentional. It signals that the patient comes before the information.

Medical Student:
I see that.

Preceptor:
Next time, I want you to try that exact sequence.

Medical Student:
Pause, eye contact, then speak.

Preceptor:
"Yes. Make the behavior visible to yourself.

Medical Student:
I'll do that.

Preceptor:
That's how it becomes repeatable.

What has been demonstrated is measurable:

- The preceptor verbalized the behavior before performing it.
- The behavior was demonstrated in real time.
- The learner was directed to observe a specific action.
- The behavior was reinforced immediately after the encounter.
- The learner was given a clear, repeatable sequence to apply.

This is making relationship behaviors visible. It transforms unconscious habits into deliberate, teachable actions that can be observed, practiced, and refined.

Example: Setting Expectations Before the Encounter

The second step is **setting expectations before encounters.** Before entering a patient room, the supervising healthcare provider can briefly frame the focus: "On this visit, pay attention to how you open the interaction and acknowledge everyone in the room." This creates a clear objective and directs the learner's attention.

Preceptor:
Before we go into this next room, let's set a clear focus.

Medical Student:
Okay.

Preceptor:
On this visit, I want you to pay attention to how the interaction begins.

Medical Student:
The introduction?

Preceptor:
Yes, specifically how you open the conversation and acknowledge everyone in the room.

Medical Student:
Got it.

Preceptor:
There will be the patient and likely a family member present.

Medical Student:
Okay.

Preceptor:
Your goal is to pause, make eye contact, greet the patient first, and then include the others.

Medical Student:
So patient first, then everyone else.

Preceptor:
Exactly.

Preceptor:
Also, remember to confirm if the patient is comfortable discussing things with others present.

Medical Student:
Right.

Preceptor:
I'm not going to focus on your medical questions this time.

Medical Student:
Just the opening.

Preceptor:
Yes. One objective.

Medical Student:
That helps.

Preceptor:
I'll observe and we'll review it right after.

Medical Student:
Okay.

Preceptor:
Take a moment before we go in. Visualize the sequence.

Medical Student:
Pause, eye contact, greet, include.

Preceptor:
Perfect. Let's go.

What has been demonstrated is measurable:

- A clear, singular objective was defined before the encounter.
- The learner's attention was directed to a specific behavior.
- The scope was intentionally narrowed to avoid overload.
- The learner verbalized the sequence before entering.
- The expectation created structure for observation and feedback.

This is setting expectations before the encounter. It transforms a routine patient visit into a focused learning opportunity with a defined and measurable goal.

Example: Assigning Specific Roles in the Encounter

The third step is **assigning specific roles.** Instead of passive observation, students should be given responsibility for defined parts of the interaction. One student may lead the introduction. Another may focus on summarizing the plan. This transforms learning from observation into participation.

Preceptor:
"Before we go into this next room, I'm going to assign each of you a specific role.

Medical Student 1:
"Okay.

Medical Student 2:
Sounds good.

Preceptor:
This way, you're both actively participating, not just observing.

Medical Student 1:
What would you like me to do?

Preceptor:
You'll lead the introduction.

Medical Student 1:
So I'll open the visit?

Preceptor:
Yes. Pause, make eye contact, greet the patient, and acknowledge anyone else in the room.

Medical Student 1:
Got it.

Preceptor (turns to 2nd student):
And you, will focus on summarizing the plan at the end.

Medical Student 2:
So I'll listen and then explain next steps?

Preceptor:
Exactly. I want you to translate the plan into clear, simple language.

Medical Student 2:
Okay.

Preceptor:
I'll guide the middle of the visit, but these parts are yours.

Medical Student 1:
That helps to know.

Medical Student 2:
Yes, it gives us something specific to focus on.

Preceptor:
Afterward, we'll review each role separately.

Medical Student 1:
Alright.

Medical Student 2:
Ready.

Preceptor:
Take a moment to think through your part.

Medical Student 1:
Introduction and acknowledgment.

Medical Student 2:
Clear summary at the end.

Preceptor:
Perfect. Let's go in.

What has been demonstrated is measurable:

- Each learner was assigned a clearly defined role.
- Responsibility replaced passive observation.
- Specific behaviors were linked to each role.
- The encounter was structured into distinct learning segments.
- Accountability and participation were increased for both learners.

This is assigning specific roles. It transforms clinical learning into active engagement, where each student contributes meaningfully and develops targeted skills within the same encounter.

Example: Real-Time Correction and Reinforcement

The fourth step is **real-time correction and reinforcement**. Feedback should occur immediately after the encounter, focusing on one or two key relational behaviors. This aligns with the principles of effective feedback: specific, timely, and actionable.

A medical student has just completed the opening of a patient encounter while the preceptor observed. As they step out of the room, the preceptor pauses in the hallway rather than moving on immediately.

Preceptor:
Let's take a moment while that's still fresh.

Medical Student:
Okay.

Preceptor:
How did that opening feel to you?

Medical Student:
I think it went okay.

Preceptor:
You did something very well.

A brief pause reinforces attention.

Preceptor:
You paused and made eye contact before speaking. That set a strong tone.

Medical Student:
I was trying to focus on that.

Preceptor:
It showed. The patient looked comfortable right away.

The positive behavior is clearly linked to impact.

Preceptor:
There's one adjustment I want you to make.

The feedback remains focused.

Medical Student:
Okay.

Preceptor:
After greeting the patient, you moved directly into questions without acknowledging the family member in the room.

Medical Student:
I didn't think about that.

Preceptor:
Next time, after greeting the patient, briefly acknowledge others with something like, "And you are?"

The correction is simple and actionable.

Medical Student:
That makes sense.

Preceptor:
So keep the pause and eye contact, and add that acknowledgment.

Medical Student:
Got it.

Preceptor:
You can apply that immediately on the next patient.

Medical Student:
I will.

Preceptor:
That's how this improves, one adjustment at a time.

What has been demonstrated is measurable:

- Feedback was delivered immediately after the encounter.
- One strength and one improvement were identified.
- The feedback was specific and behavior based.
- A clear replacement action was provided.
- The learner can apply the correction in the next interaction.

This is real-time correction and reinforcement. It ensures that learning is immediate, focused, and directly connected to observable behavior.

Example: Structured Repetition Across Clinical Settings

The fifth step is **structured repetition across settings.** Relationship skills should be practiced not only in one rotation, but across all clinical environments, outpatient, inpatient, emergency, and specialty care. Consistency across contexts reinforces that these skills are universal, not situational.

A medical student is rotating through different clinical environments over several weeks. The same relational skill, opening the encounter with presence and eye contact, is reinforced across each setting.

Outpatient Clinic

Preceptor:
Before we go in, remember your opening sequence.

Medical Student:
Pause, eye contact, greet first.

Preceptor:
Exactly.

(After the visit)

Preceptor:
You held eye contact well. Keep reinforcing that.

Inpatient Ward

Preceptor:
Even in the hospital, the same rule applies. Slow down your entry.

Medical Student:
Even if it's busy?

Preceptor:
Especially then.

(After the encounter)

Preceptor:
You rushed slightly. Reset and try again on the next patient.

Emergency Department

Preceptor:
This environment is fast, but your opening still matters.

Medical Student:
I'll keep it consistent.

Preceptor:
Good. Even a brief pause changes the interaction.

(Afterward)

Preceptor:
That was better. You created connection quickly.

Specialty Clinic

Preceptor:
Different setting, same expectation.

Medical Student:
Pause, eye contact, greet.

Preceptor:
Yes. It should feel automatic now.

(After the visit)

Preceptor:
That's becoming natural for you.

Medical Student:
It's starting to feel the same everywhere.

Preceptor:
That's the goal.

Medical Student:
Not dependent on the setting.

Preceptor:
Exactly. Consistency creates habit.

What has been demonstrated is measurable:

- The same behavior was reinforced across multiple clinical environments.
- Expectations remained consistent despite differences in setting and pace.
- Feedback was repeated and refined over time.
- The learner practiced the same skill under varying conditions.
- The behavior began to transition from effort to habit.

This is structured repetition across settings. It ensures that relationship skills are not situational, but universal, becoming a reliable and consistent part of clinical practice regardless of environment.

Example: Evaluation Alongside Clinical Competence

The sixth step is **evaluation alongside clinical competence.** Relationship behaviors should be assessed with the same rigor as diagnostic ability. When learners know they are being evaluated on how they communicate and connect, those behaviors become integral to their performance.

A medical student has just completed a patient encounter involving both history-taking and explanation of a treatment plan. The preceptor and student step aside to review the performance.

Preceptor:
Let's go through this the same way we evaluate all encounters.

Medical Student:
Okay.

Preceptor:
First, your clinical reasoning. You identified the likely diagnosis correctly and asked the right follow-up questions.

Medical Student:
Good.

Preceptor:
Now, I'm going to evaluate your communication with the same level of detail.

The expectation is clearly equal.

Medical Student:
Alright.

Preceptor:
When you entered the room, you went straight to the computer before making eye contact.

Medical Student:
I didn't notice that.

Preceptor:
That affects how the patient perceives the interaction from the start

The behavior is assessed with the same precision as a clinical finding.

Preceptor:
Next, during your explanation, you used the term 'inflammation' without clarifying what that means.

Medical Student:
I see.

Preceptor:
The patient nodded but did not demonstrate a clear understanding.

Medical Student:
So I should simplify that?

Preceptor:
Yes. Just as you refine a diagnosis, you refine how you explain it.

The parallel is made explicit.

Preceptor:
Both your clinical reasoning and your communication are part of your performance.

Medical Student:
That makes sense.

Preceptor:
You wouldn't accept being imprecise in diagnosis. The same standard applies here.

Medical Student:
I understand.

Preceptor:
On your next patient, I'll be evaluating both again.

Medical Student:
I'll focus on both.

What has been demonstrated is measurable:

- Communication was evaluated alongside clinical reasoning.
- Specific relational behaviors were identified and assessed.
- The same level of rigor was applied to both domains.
- The learner understood that communication is not secondary.
- Performance expectations were aligned across clinical and relational skills.

This is an evaluation alongside clinical competence. It ensures that how a healthcare provider connects with patients is held to the same standard as how they diagnose and treat, making both inseparable parts of quality care.

Finally, integration requires **role modeling at every level.** Students learn as much from what is demonstrated as from what is taught. When attending healthcare providers consistently exhibit presence, clarity, and relational awareness, those behaviors become the standard.

When relationship training is fully integrated into clinical rotations, it ceases to be an abstract concept. It becomes part of the identity of the healthcare provider in training, because clinical excellence is not only defined by what is known, but by how that knowledge is delivered, perceived, and experienced in the room.

Part VI

A Practical Framework for Daily Practice

Chapter 23	The 5-Step Interaction Model	272
Chapter 24	Micro-Skills That Make a Major Difference	281
Chapter 25	What Patients Remember Most	286
Chapter 26	Repairing a Damaged Interaction	290
Chapter 27	The 10-Second Orientation Rule	298
Chapter 28	The Waiting Room Problem	303
Chapter 29	Setting the Patient's Expectations — The Process Explained	310

Chapter 23

The 5-Step Interaction Model

A Repeatable Structure for Patient Encounters

In clinical practice, consistency is what transforms good intentions into reliable outcomes. While every patient encounter is unique, the structure that supports those encounters should not be left to chance. A clear, repeatable model allows healthcare providers to navigate complexity without losing presence, clarity, or control.

The 5-Step Interaction Model provides a simple, dependable framework that can be applied across all clinical settings. It does not restrict individuality. It supports it. By creating a consistent structure, it allows the healthcare provider to focus more fully on the patient rather than on what comes next.

Step 1: Establish Presence

The encounter begins before a single word is spoken. The healthcare provider pauses, makes eye contact, and acknowledges everyone in the room. This step sets the tone. It communicates awareness, respect, and professionalism within the first few seconds.

The healthcare provider stands just outside the exam room door, briefly still, taking a moment to reset before entering. There is no rush in the movement that follows. The healthcare provider enters the room without looking at the chart or computer. The healthcare provider pauses briefly, lifts their gaze and makes direct eye contact with the patient before speaking.

Provider:
Good morning.

The tone is calm, grounded, and unhurried. Eye contact is maintained for a moment, allowing the greeting to register.

Provider:
Hi, I'm Dr. Harris. It's nice to meet you.

The healthcare provider then shifts attention naturally to others in the room.

Provider:
And you are?

Family Member:
I'm her mother.

The healthcare provider nods slightly.

Provider:
Thank you for being here.

The healthcare provider briefly acknowledges each person present with eye contact, then returns primary focus to the patient. Posture remains open, shoulders oriented toward the patient, with no immediate movement toward the computer or chart. No interruption. No divided attention. The first several seconds are fully directed toward the people in the room. The entire sequence takes less than ten seconds.

What has been demonstrated is measurable:

- Eye contact is established before speaking.
- The patient is greeted before engaging with any tools or data.
- All individuals in the room are acknowledged.
- Body orientation is directed toward the patient.
- There is no chart or computer interaction during the opening moments

This is establishing presence. It is a deliberate, repeatable sequence that defines the tone of the encounter before any clinical discussion begins.

Step 2: Invite the Patient's Narrative

The healthcare provider opens with an open-ended prompt such as, "Tell me what's been going on." The patient is allowed to speak without interruption. This step ensures that the patient's perspective leads the encounter, not the healthcare provider's assumptions.

The healthcare provider has established presence and now transitions into the patient's story without redirecting or narrowing the conversation prematurely. The healthcare provider maintains eye contact, posture oriented toward the patient, with no attention to the computer.

Provider:
Tell me what's been going on.

The question is open, neutral, and unhurried. A brief silence follows. The healthcare provider does not fill the space.

Patient:
I've been having this pressure in my chest for the past few days.

The healthcare provider nods slightly, signaling attention without interruption.

Patient:
At first it only happened when I was walking, but now I feel it even when I'm sitting.

The healthcare provider remains still, listening. No interruption. No redirection.

Patient:
It's starting to worry me because it doesn't seem to be going away.

The healthcare provider allows the patient to complete the thought fully. A brief pause.

Provider:
Go on.

The invitation is subtle, encouraging continuation.

Patient:
I also feel a little short of breath sometimes.

The healthcare provider continues to listen, maintaining presence. Only after the patient naturally pauses does the healthcare provider respond.

Provider:
You've been feeling chest pressure for a few days, and now it's happening even at rest, along with some shortness of breath.

The healthcare provider reflects the narrative, demonstrating understanding.

Patient:
Yes, exactly.

The patient feels heard and validated.

What has been demonstrated is measurable:

- An open-ended prompt was used to initiate the narrative.
- The patient was allowed to speak without interruption.
- The healthcare provider maintained full attention and presence throughout.

- Silence was used appropriately to allow the patient to continue.
- The healthcare provider reflected back key elements to confirm understanding.

This is inviting the patient's narrative. It ensures that the encounter begins with the patient's perspective, creating a foundation of understanding before clinical direction is introduced.

Step 3: Structure and Clarify

After the initial narrative, the healthcare provider begins to guide the conversation with focused questions. Information is organized, gaps are addressed, and key details are clarified. This step balances openness with clinical direction.

The patient has completed their initial narrative. The healthcare provider now shifts from open listening to guided clarification, maintaining a calm and organized approach.

Provider:
Thank you for explaining that. I'm going to ask a few specific questions to better understand what's going on.

The transition is explicit and respectful.

Patient:
Okay.

Provider:
You mentioned the pressure started a few days ago. Do you remember exactly when it began?

Patient:
About three days ago.

Provider:
And when it first started, was it only with activity like walking?

Patient:
"Yes, only when I was moving.

Provider:
Now you're feeling it even at rest, correct?

Patient:
Yes.

The healthcare provider organizes the timeline.

Provider:
On a scale from 1 to 10, how intense is the pressure when it's at its worst?

Patient:
Maybe a 6.

Provider:
Does it spread anywhere, like your arm, jaw, or back?

Patient:
No, it stays in my chest.

Provider:
Any nausea, sweating, or dizziness with it?

Patient:
A little shortness of breath, but no nausea.

The healthcare provider systematically addresses key clinical elements.

Provider:
Have you noticed anything that makes it better or worse?

Patient:
It gets worse when I walk.

Provider:
Have you experienced anything like this before?

Patient:
No.

The healthcare provider briefly summarizes to ensure accuracy.

Provider:
So this started three days ago with activity, now occurs at rest, is about a 6 out of 10, and is associated with some shortness of breath but no spreading pain.

Patient:
Yes, that's right.

The structure is clear, organized, and complete.

What has been demonstrated is measurable:

- The healthcare provider clearly transitioned from open narrative to focused questioning.
- Questions were organized to establish a timeline, severity, and associated symptoms.
- Gaps in information were identified and addressed.
- The healthcare provider maintained clarity without rushing or overwhelming the patient.
- A summary was used to confirm accuracy and alignment.

This is structure and clarification. It transforms the patient's narrative into clinically meaningful information while preserving clarity, organization, and control of the encounter.

Step 4: Explain and Align

The healthcare provider explains findings and next steps in clear, understandable language. The plan is presented in a structured way, and the patient's understanding is confirmed. This step ensures that information is not only delivered, but received.

The healthcare provider has gathered and clarified the necessary information and now transitions into explanation. The healthcare provider pauses briefly, making eye contact to ensure the patient is ready to receive information.

Provider:
I'm going to explain what I think is happening, and then we'll go over what we do next.

The structure is stated clearly.

Patient:
Okay.

Provider:
Based on your symptoms and exam, this does not appear to be coming from your heart.

The healthcare provider begins with a clear, direct statement. The patient visibly relaxes.

Provider:
Instead, it's most consistent with irritation of the muscles in your chest. That can cause pressure, especially when you move.

Medical language is translated into understandable terms.

Patient:
So it's not something serious?

Provider:
It's not dangerous, but I understand why it felt concerning.

The healthcare provider acknowledges both the clinical and emotional perspectives. The healthcare provider continues in a structured format.

Provider:
Here's the plan. First, I'll recommend a medication to reduce the inflammation. Second, I want you to avoid heavy activity for a few days. Third, if the symptoms change or worsen, you should contact us right away.

The steps are clearly organized and paced. The healthcare provider pauses.

Provider:
Can you tell me, in your own words, what the plan is?

Patient:
It's muscle-related. I take the medication, rest, and call if it gets worse.

Provider:
Exactly.

The healthcare provider confirms understanding.

Provider:
What questions do you have?

Patient:
No, that makes sense.

The patient demonstrates alignment.

What has been demonstrated is measurable:

- Information was explained in clear, non-technical language.
- The explanation followed a structured sequence.
- Emotional concerns were acknowledged alongside clinical facts.
- The patient was asked to repeat the plan to confirm understanding.
- Questions were invited to ensure alignment.

This is explained and aligned. It ensures that information is not only delivered, but understood, accepted, and integrated into the patient's next steps.

Step 5: Close with Confirmation and Support

The encounter ends with alignment. The healthcare provider confirms understanding, invites final questions, and reinforces availability for follow-up. The closing is intentional, not rushed, ensuring the patient leaves with clarity and confidence.

The clinical discussion has concluded, and the healthcare provider transitions deliberately into the closing phase, maintaining full presence. The healthcare provider remains seated, facing the patient, with steady eye contact.

Provider:
Before we finish, I want to make sure everything is clear.

The tone is calm and unhurried.

Patient:
Okay.

Provider:
Can you walk me through your understanding of what's going on and what the plan is?

The request is open and respectful.

Patient:
It's not my heart, it's muscle-related. I'll take the medication, rest, and call if anything changes.

The healthcare provider nods.

Provider:
That's exactly right.

A brief pause allows space for additional thoughts.

Provider:
What questions do you still have?

The phrasing assumes there may be questions, encouraging openness.

Patient:
I think I'm okay.

The healthcare provider does not rush.

Provider:
Is there anything we didn't talk about that you were hoping to address today?

This creates a final opportunity for missed concerns.

Patient:
No, I feel good about it.

The healthcare provider acknowledges both understanding and reassurance.

Provider:
I'm glad. You did the right thing coming in.

The healthcare provider reinforces the patient's decision.

Provider:
If anything changes or you feel uncertain, please reach out. We're here for you.

Support is made explicit. The healthcare provider maintains eye contact for a final moment before standing.

Provider:
Take care of yourself. We'll follow up as planned.

The encounter ends with clarity, support, and confidence.

What has been demonstrated is measurable:

- Understanding was confirmed through patient explanation.
- Final questions were invited in an open and supportive way.
- Additional concerns were proactively explored.
- Reassurance and continued support were clearly communicated.
- The closing was deliberate, not rushed.

This is closing with confirmation and support. It ensures that the patient leaves not only informed, but confident, supported, and fully aligned with the plan of care.

This model is not theoretical. It is practical and repeatable. It can be applied in a routine visit, a complex consultation, or a high-pressure environment. With repetition, it becomes internalized, allowing the healthcare provider to move through each step naturally, because in medicine, variability in patients is inevitable; variability in structure does not have to be. A consistent interaction model creates reliability, and reliability is what patients experience as trust.

Chapter 24

Micro-Skills That Make a Major Difference

Eye Contact, Pauses, Tone, and Body Language

In clinical practice, it is often assumed that outcomes are driven primarily by knowledge, diagnosis, and treatment decisions. While these are essential, they are not what patients experience first, nor what they remember most. What shapes the patient's perception of care in real time are the smallest, most immediate behaviors: where the healthcare provider looks, how long they pause, the tone of their voice, and the way they position their body in the room.

These are micro-skills. They are subtle, often unconscious, and frequently overlooked. Yet they carry disproportionate influence.

The First Signal of Presence

Eye contact is one of the most powerful signals of presence. It communicates attention, respect, and engagement without a single word. When established early and maintained appropriately, it reassures the patient that they are being seen and prioritized. When absent, even briefly, it can create a sense of distance or disinterest.

Eye contact is not simply a social courtesy. In a clinical setting, it is one of the earliest and most influential signals a patient receives. Before a diagnosis is formed, before a question is asked, the patient is already interpreting whether they are being seen, valued, and prioritized. Eye contact is often the first indicator.

When a healthcare provider establishes eye contact immediately upon entering the room, it creates an instant shift in the environment. It communicates, without words, *"I am here with you."* This moment, often lasting only a second or two, sets the tone for everything that follows. It anchors the interaction in presence rather than process.

The timing of eye contact matters. When it occurs before the healthcare provider looks at a chart, computer, or notes, it signals that the patient comes first. When it is delayed, even briefly, the opposite message can be perceived: that the task takes precedence over the person. Patients are highly attuned to this distinction, even if they cannot articulate it.

Equally important is the quality of eye contact. It should be natural, steady, and unforced. It is not about staring or maintaining continuous gaze, but about returning to the patient consistently throughout the interaction. This rhythm, looking, listening, briefly shifting, and returning, creates a sense of engagement and attentiveness.

Eye contact also functions as a regulator of conversation. When a healthcare provider maintains appropriate eye contact while listening, patients are more likely to continue speaking, to expand on their thoughts, and to share details they might otherwise withhold. When eye contact is absent, patients often shorten their responses, unsure if the healthcare provider is fully engaged.

There is also an emotional dimension. In moments of concern, uncertainty, or vulnerability, patients look for nonverbal reassurance. Eye contact provides that reassurance. It conveys steadiness, confidence, and attention in a way that words alone cannot.

Conversely, the absence of eye contact carries weight. Looking at a screen, writing continuously, or focusing elsewhere during key moments can unintentionally communicate disinterest or distraction. Even brief lapses, especially at the beginning of an encounter, can create a subtle sense of distance that is difficult to reverse.

What makes eye contact particularly powerful is that it requires no additional time. It is not an added task. It is a shift in attention.

It is also measurable and teachable. A healthcare provider can be trained to establish eye contact within the first few seconds of entering the room, to maintain it during key parts of the conversation, and to return to it after brief interruptions. With repetition, it becomes automatic.

In the end, eye contact is not about technique. It is about alignment. It ensures that the healthcare provider's attention is directed where it matters most, toward the person in front of them, because before patients assess what is said, they perceive whether they are being seen.

The Space That Reveals Meaning

Pauses create space. In conversation, silence is often avoided, but in medicine, it is essential. A well-timed pause allows the patient to think, to continue, or to process information. It prevents the healthcare provider from rushing ahead and missing critical details. Pauses are not empty moments. They are active opportunities for connection.

In most conversations, silence is uncomfortable. It is often interpreted as hesitation, uncertainty, or a break in momentum. As a result, people instinctively fill it. In medicine, this instinct can quietly interfere with understanding.

A well-timed pause is not a gap. It is a deliberate act. When a healthcare provider asks a question and immediately follows it with another, or begins to rephrase before the patient has had time to respond, the patient's thought process is interrupted. What might have been a fuller, more meaningful answer becomes shortened or lost entirely. The absence of pauses compresses the patient's voice.

When a pause is allowed, something different happens. After a question is asked, a brief silence gives the patient time to organize their thoughts. Many patients do not present their concerns in a linear or immediate way. They reflect, search for words, and decide what feels important enough to say. Without space, that process is cut short. With space, it unfolds.

Pauses also signal permission. When a healthcare provider asks, "Tell me what's been going on," and then remains still and attentive, the silence that follows communicates, *"You can take your time."* This often leads to richer, more complete narratives. Patients may begin with surface details, pause, and then continue with something more significant. That second layer is frequently where the most important information resides.

There is also a role for pauses after information is given. When a healthcare provider explains a diagnosis or outlines a plan, patients need time to process what they have heard. Without a pause, the information becomes a continuous stream, difficult to absorb. With a pause, the patient can reflect, formulate questions, and engage more meaningfully.

Pauses are equally powerful in emotional moments. When a patient expresses fear, uncertainty, or distress, the immediate impulse may be to respond quickly with reassurance or solutions. Yet a brief pause, combined with presence, often communicates more. It allows the patient's experience to be acknowledged without interruption or minimization.

Importantly, pauses are not passive. They require control. The healthcare provider remains attentive, maintains eye contact, and resists the urge to fill the silence. This transforms the pause from absence into engagement.

Like other micro-skills, pauses are measurable and trainable. A healthcare provider can learn to wait two to three seconds after asking a question before speaking again. They can become aware of moments where they typically interrupt silence and choose instead to allow it. These are small adjustments, but they have a cumulative effect, because in the space where nothing is said, patients often say the most.

The Carrier of Meaning

Tone of voice shapes how information is received. The same words can either reassure or alarm, depending on how they are delivered. A calm, steady tone conveys control and confidence. A rushed or distracted tone can create anxiety, even if the content is accurate. Patients respond not only to what is said, but to how it sounds.

In clinical communication, words are only part of the message. Tone is what gives those words direction, weight, and emotional context. Two healthcare providers can say the exact same sentence, and yet the patient may leave with entirely different impressions based on how it was delivered.

A calm, steady tone communicates control. It signals that the healthcare provider is composed, attentive, and confident in their approach. Patients often interpret this as safety. Even when discussing something uncertain or complex, a measured tone reassures the patient that the situation is being handled with clarity and care.

In contrast, a rushed or fragmented tone can introduce unease. When speech is rapid, clipped, or distracted, patients may sense urgency or disorganization, even if none is intended. The content may be accurate, but the delivery creates tension. Patients begin to wonder if something is being missed, overlooked, or minimized.

Tone also influences how patients interpret information emotionally. For example, saying, "We'll need to run a few more tests," in a neutral, steady tone feels different from saying the same words quickly or with hesitation. The first conveys thoughtful planning. The second can suggest concern or uncertainty. The difference is not in the words, but in how they sound.

There is also a relational aspect to tone. A warm, attentive tone communicates presence. It suggests that the healthcare provider is not simply delivering information but engaging with the patient. This does not require exaggerated friendliness or artificial softness. It requires alignment between intention and delivery.

Tone becomes especially important in moments of explanation and reassurance. When patients are anxious, they listen not only for information, but for cues about how to feel. A grounded tone can reduce anxiety without explicitly addressing it. It creates a sense of steadiness that patients often mirror.

Like other micro-skills, tone can be adjusted deliberately: a healthcare provider can slow their pace slightly, they can allow space between sentences, or they can avoid speaking while turning away or multitasking. These small adjustments refine how the message is received.

Tone is not an accessory to communication. It is part of the message itself, because patients do not separate what they hear from how it is said. They experience both at the same time, and often, it is the tone that stays with them longest.

Body Language: The Unspoken Alignment

Body language reinforces or contradicts everything else. Orientation matters. A healthcare provider who faces the patient fully, sits when appropriate, and maintains an open posture signals availability and attention. Turning away, standing at a distance, or focusing on a screen sends the opposite message, often unintentionally.

Body language is constant. It is present before words, during conversation, and even in silence. In a clinical setting, it either reinforces what the healthcare provider is saying or quietly contradicts it. Patients may not consciously analyze these signals, but they respond to them immediately.

Orientation is the foundation. When a healthcare provider faces the patient, shoulders aligned and body directed toward them, it conveys attention and availability. It says, without words, *"You have my focus."* This alignment creates a sense of connection that supports everything else in the interaction.

Sitting, when appropriate, further strengthens this signal. It reduces perceived hierarchy, slows the pace of the encounter, and conveys that time is being given intentionally. Even brief moments seated can change how the interaction is experienced.

Posture also matters. An open posture, arms relaxed, body slightly leaning forward, suggests engagement and receptiveness. It invites conversation. In contrast, crossed arms, turning partially away, or maintaining physical distance can create subtle barriers. These positions may be unintentional, but they can be perceived as disinterest or detachment.

Movement within the room carries meaning as well. Turning toward a computer while the patient is speaking, even briefly, shifts attention away from the patient. Repeated movements like this fragment the interaction. The patient begins to compete with other focal points in the room.

Similarly, standing near the door or maintaining distance can signal urgency or an impending exit, even if the healthcare provider intends to stay. Patients often interpret positioning as an indication of how much time or attention they will receive.

Body language becomes especially important during moments of listening. A still, attentive posture communicates that the healthcare provider is fully present. Small gestures, such as nodding or slight forward movement, reinforce that the patient is being heard. These are not performative actions. They are physical expressions of attention.

Like other micro-skills, body language is adjustable. A healthcare provider can choose to orient fully before speaking. They can sit rather than stand when appropriate. They can become aware of where their body is directed during key moments. These are simple changes, but they have an immediate impact.

Body language does not require additional time or effort. It requires awareness, because in every interaction, the healthcare provider is communicating twice: once through words, and once through presence.

When those two are aligned, trust is strengthened. When they are not, patients notice the difference, even if it is never spoken.

What makes these micro-skills so important is that they occur continuously throughout the encounter. They are not isolated actions. They are ongoing signals that shape the patient's experience moment by moment.

They are also measurable and trainable. A healthcare provider can learn to establish eye contact within the first few seconds of entering the room. They can learn to pause after asking a question rather than filling the silence. They can become aware of their tone and adjust it deliberately. They can position their body in a way that supports connection rather than distraction.

These adjustments require awareness, not additional time, and that is the critical point. Micro-skills do not slow down care. They improve it without extending it. When practiced consistently, they become automatic. When they become automatic, they define presence, because in the patient's experience, care is not only delivered through decisions. It is communicated through behavior, moment by moment, often in ways that are never spoken but always felt.

Chapter 25

What Patients Remember Most

Moments That Define Care

Patients rarely remember every detail of a clinical encounter. They may not recall the exact terminology used, the sequence of questions asked, or even the specifics of the physical exam. What they do remember are moments. Brief, often subtle interactions that shape how the entire experience is perceived.

These moments are not accidental. They occur at predictable points in the encounter, and they carry disproportionate weight.

Patient Testimonials: The Moment of Entry

The first is **the moment of entry.** When the healthcare provider walks into the room, patients form an immediate impression. Did the healthcare provider look at them? Did they feel acknowledged? Was there a pause, or a sense of rushing? Within seconds, patients begin to decide whether they feel seen or overlooked.

Testimonial 1:

"When the doctor walked in, the first thing I noticed was that he stopped, looked directly at me, and said my name. It sounds simple, but it made me feel like I mattered right away. I wasn't just the next appointment. I felt seen before we even started talking."

Testimonial 2:

"The doctor came in quickly, already looking down at the computer, and started asking questions without really looking at me. Nothing he said was wrong, but something felt off. I didn't feel connected to him. It was like I was part of a process instead of a person in the room."

Testimonial 3:

"She walked in, paused for a second, and made eye contact with me and my husband before saying anything. That moment stuck with me. It felt calm, not rushed. I remember thinking, 'Okay, she's really here with us.' It changed how I felt about the entire visit."

Patient Testimonials: The Moment of Listening

The second is **the moment of listening.** Patients remember whether they were allowed to speak. They recall if they were interrupted, or if there was space to express what mattered to them. Even a brief interruption early in the conversation can define the entire interaction in their memory.

Testimonial 1:

"He asked me what was going on and then just listened. He didn't interrupt, didn't rush me. I actually paused at one point, and he waited. That made me feel like what I was saying mattered. I ended up sharing things I wasn't even planning to mention."

Testimonial 2:

"I barely got two sentences out before the doctor started asking more questions and redirecting me. I understand they're trying to be efficient, but I left feeling like I didn't fully explain what was wrong. It stayed with me more than anything else from the visit."

Testimonial 3:

"She let me talk. Really talk. There were a couple of moments where I stopped, and instead of jumping in, she just gave me space. That's when I said what was actually worrying me. I don't remember everything she said after, but I remember that she listened."

Patient Testimonials: The Moment of Understanding

The third is **the moment of understanding.** When a healthcare provider reflects back what the patient has said, accurately and clearly, it creates a powerful sense of validation. Patients remember feeling understood far more than they remember the exact questions that led there.

Testimonial 1:

"After I explained everything, the doctor repeated it back to me in a way that made me feel like he really got it. He said it more clearly than I could. In that moment, I felt understood, not just heard. That stayed with me."

Testimonial 2:

"I talked for a while, but the doctor just moved on to the next question without really acknowledging what I said. It made me feel like maybe I hadn't explained it well, or that it didn't matter. I left unsure if he truly understood my concern."

Testimonial 3:

"She listened and then said, 'So what I'm hearing is…' and explained it back to me. It was exactly what I meant, even the part I struggled to say. That moment made me trust her. I felt like we were on the same page."

Patient Testimonials: The Moment of Explanation

The fourth is **the moment of explanation.** Clarity matters. Patients remember whether the explanation made sense to them. They recall if it reduced their anxiety or increased it. The tone, pacing, and simplicity of the explanation often matter more than the technical details.

Testimonial 1:

"When the doctor explained what was going on, he used simple terms and took his time. I remember feeling my anxiety go down as he spoke. It wasn't just what he said; it was how clearly and calmly he said it. I left feeling like I understood everything."

Testimonial 2:

"The explanation was full of medical terms I didn't really understand. I nodded, but honestly, I was confused. I didn't want to keep asking questions. I left more anxious than when I came in because I wasn't sure what was actually wrong."

Testimonial 3:

"She explained everything step by step and then paused to make sure I understood. That pause made a difference. I felt comfortable asking a question I might have kept to myself. It made the whole situation feel manageable instead of overwhelming."

Patient Testimonials: The Moment of Reassurance or Uncertainty

The fifth is **the moment of reassurance or uncertainty.** In situations where there is concern, patients remember how the healthcare provider handled it. Did they feel guided? Did they feel dismissed? These emotional impressions often stay with them long after the visit.

Testimonial 1:

"I remember telling the doctor how worried I was, and instead of brushing it off, he slowed down and explained things clearly. He didn't promise everything was fine, but he gave me a plan and stayed calm. That made me feel like I wasn't facing it alone."

Testimonial 2:

"When I shared my concerns, the doctor quickly said, 'It's nothing to worry about,' and moved on. I know it was meant to reassure me, but it felt like my fears weren't taken seriously. I left feeling dismissed and still anxious."

Testimonial 3:

"She was honest that we didn't have all the answers yet, but the way she said it mattered. She explained what we knew, what we were still figuring out, and what the next steps were. I didn't feel uncertain; I felt supported through the uncertainty."

What is striking is that these moments are not complex. They are brief, repeatable, and within the health-care provider's control. Yet they shape the patient's perception more than any single clinical decision.

This does not diminish the importance of medical accuracy. It highlights that accuracy alone is not what patients carry with them. They carry the experience. And that experience is built not from the entirety of the visit, but from a series of defining moments that signal whether they were seen, heard, understood, and cared for, because in the end, patients may not remember everything that was said, but they remember how they felt in the presence of the person who said it.

Chapter 26

Repairing a Damaged Interaction

How to Recover When Things Go Wrong

Even the most skilled clinicians will have moments where an interaction does not go as intended. A patient feels interrupted. A comment is perceived as dismissive. The healthcare provider becomes rushed or distracted. These moments are not rare. They are inevitable. What defines quality of care is not the absence of missteps, but the ability to recognize and repair them.

Example: Step 1—Awareness in Repairing an Interaction

The first step in repair is awareness. Something shifts in the room. The patient becomes quieter, more guarded, or visibly frustrated. The tone changes. These signals are often subtle, but they are present. Recognizing them in real time is the foundation of recovery.

The healthcare provider is midway through the encounter, asking follow-up questions after the patient's initial explanation.

Provider:
How long has the pain been going on?

Patient:
About a week, but it's not just the pain, it's—

Provider:
Any nausea or vomiting?

The healthcare provider redirects quickly. The patient pauses.

Patient:
No... not really.

The tone shifts. The patient's posture changes slightly, shoulders pulling inward. Eye contact decreases. Responses become shorter.

Provider:
Any changes in appetite?

Patient:
No.

A brief silence follows. The healthcare provider notices something different. The energy in the room has changed. The patient is no longer expanding, only answering.

The healthcare provider pauses. Instead of continuing with the next question, the healthcare provider looks directly at the patient, observing. There is a subtle recognition: the patient had more to say and was interrupted. The patient's expression appears slightly withdrawn.

The healthcare provider does not move forward immediately. The awareness is internal but clear. The healthcare provider shifts posture, turning fully toward the patient again. A moment of stillness. The encounter has not yet been repaired, but the healthcare provider has recognized the shift.

What has been demonstrated is measurable:

- A change in patient behavior was observed (shorter answers, reduced eye contact).
- A shift in tone and engagement was recognized.
- The healthcare provider paused instead of continuing automatically.
- Attention was redirected back to the patient.
- The moment of disruption was identified in real time.

This is awareness. It is the point at which the healthcare provider recognizes that something in the interaction has changed, creating the opportunity for repair before the distance becomes permanent.

Example: Step 2—Pause and Reset in Repairing an Interaction

The second step is to pause and reset. Rather than continuing forward, the healthcare provider deliberately slows down. This may be as simple as stopping mid-sentence, reestablishing eye contact, and redirecting attention fully back to the patient. The pause itself signals that something is being acknowledged.

The healthcare provider has just recognized a shift in the patient's engagement. The patient has become quieter, offering brief responses after being interrupted.

Provider:
Any changes in your appetite or sleep—

The healthcare provider stops mid-sentence. A brief pause. The healthcare provider lifts their gaze fully from their notes and reestablishes direct eye contact with the patient. The body shifts slightly, turning fully toward the patient. Silence is allowed for a moment. The pace of the encounter slows.

Provider:
"Let me pause for a second."

The tone is calm and grounded. Another brief silence. The healthcare provider remains still, attentive, and present. The patient looks back up, noticing the shift. The healthcare provider does not immediately resume questioning. Instead, the focus is clearly redirected. The interruption of momentum is intentional.

The healthcare provider's posture is open, no longer angled toward the computer or chart. The room feels quieter, more centered. The patient's expression softens slightly. The healthcare provider maintains eye contact, signaling readiness to listen. No new questions are introduced yet. The pause itself becomes the intervention.

What has been demonstrated is measurable:

- The healthcare provider stopped mid-pattern instead of continuing automatically.
- Eye contact was deliberately reestablished.
- Body orientation shifted fully back to the patient.
- The pace of the interaction slowed noticeably.
- Silence was used to signal acknowledgment and reset attention.

This is a pause and a reset. It creates a clear break in the previous interaction pattern, signaling to the patient that the healthcare provider is aware, present, and ready to re-engage before moving forward.

Example: Step 3—Naming the Moment in Repairing an Interaction

The third step is naming the moment. This is where many clinicians hesitate, yet it is one of the most powerful actions. A brief, direct statement such as, "I feel like I may have interrupted you earlier," or "I want to make sure I'm understanding you correctly," brings the issue into the open without defensiveness.

The healthcare provider has paused and reset. The room is quieter, attention restored. Now comes the moment many clinicians avoid. The healthcare provider maintains eye contact, tone steady and neutral.

Provider:
I want to take a moment here.

A brief pause.

Provider:
I think I may have interrupted you earlier when you were explaining what you were feeling.

The statement is direct, without defensiveness or justification. The patient looks up, slightly surprised, then nods.

Patient:
Yeah… I was trying to explain something.

The healthcare provider does not rush to correct or move past it.

Provider:
I want to make sure I understand you fully.

The focus remains on the patient, not the healthcare provider. A brief silence follows. The patient's posture shifts, becoming more open again.

Patient:
It wasn't just the pain… it was also how suddenly it started.

The healthcare provider listens, allowing the patient to re-enter the narrative. There is no over explanation, no apology layered with justification. The moment has been acknowledged clearly and simply. The tension in the room decreases. The patient resumes speaking more naturally. The healthcare provider maintains steady eye contact, fully present.

What has been demonstrated is measurable:

- The healthcare provider explicitly named the disruption in the interaction.
- The statement was brief, clear, and non-defensive.
- Responsibility was implied without overexplaining.
- The patient was given space to respond and re-engage.
- The interaction shifted back toward openness and trust.

This is naming the moment. It brings an unspoken disruption into the open, allowing it to be addressed directly and respectfully, which is often the turning point in repairing the interaction.

Example: Step 4—Taking Responsibility Without Over explanation

The fourth step is taking responsibility without over explanation. A simple acknowledgment is often enough: "I'm sorry, I should have let you finish." This is not about self-justification. It is about restoring trust. Overexplaining can dilute the sincerity of the moment.

The healthcare provider has already named the moment. The patient has indicated they were interrupted. The room is attentive and quiet. The healthcare provider maintains eye contact, tone steady and composed.

Provider:
I'm sorry, I should have let you finish.

The statement is brief and direct. No added justification. No explanation of time pressure or workflow. The healthcare provider remains still. A short pause follows. The patient nods.

Patient:
I was trying to explain how it started.

The healthcare provider listens without interrupting. There is no attempt to regain control of the conversation prematurely. The responsibility has been taken, and space is allowed. The healthcare provider's posture remains open, fully oriented toward the patient. No shift back to the computer. No distraction. The patient continues speaking.

Patient:
It came on suddenly, and that's what scared me.

The healthcare provider listens, nodding slightly. The interaction begins to feel more balanced again. The apology stands on its own, without being diluted. The patient's tone becomes more natural. Trust begins to reestablish.

What has been demonstrated is measurable:

- A clear acknowledgment of the misstep was made.
- The statement was brief and free of justification.
- No defensive language or explanation was added.
- The healthcare provider allowed space after the acknowledgment.
- The patient resumed speaking with increased openness.

This is taking responsibility without over explanation. It restores trust through clarity and sincerity, allowing the interaction to move forward without unnecessary distraction or dilution of the moment.

Example: Step 5—Reinviting the Patient's Voice

The fifth step is reinviting the patient's voice. After acknowledging the misstep, the healthcare provider must create space again: "Please go ahead, I want to hear the rest of what you were saying." This signals that the patient's perspective remains central.

The healthcare provider has acknowledged the interruption and taken responsibility. The room has settled, but the interaction is not complete until the patient is fully brought back into the conversation. The healthcare provider maintains eye contact, posture open and directed toward the patient. There is a brief pause.

Provider:
Please go ahead. I want to hear the rest of what you were saying.

The tone is calm, genuine, and unhurried. The invitation is clear. The healthcare provider does not add additional questions or redirect. Silence is allowed. The patient looks up, reassessing the space.

Patient:
It started suddenly… I was just sitting, and then I felt this pressure.

The healthcare provider nods slightly, listening. No interruption.

Patient:
That's what worried me. It didn't feel like something that built up.

The healthcare provider maintains steady eye contact, allowing the patient to continue fully. The patient's voice becomes more fluid.

Patient:
I think that's why I got anxious about it.

The healthcare provider remains still, attentive. The narrative resumes naturally, without fragmentation. The earlier disruption has been repaired through reinitiation. The patient is no longer guarded. The healthcare provider does not rush forward. The space remains open until the patient completes their thought.

What has been demonstrated is measurable:

- The healthcare provider explicitly invited the patient to continue.
- The invitation was clear, simple, and patient-centered.
- Silence was used to allow re-engagement.
- The patient resumed a fuller, more complete narrative.
- The interaction returned to a balanced and open exchange.

This is reinviting the patient's voice. It ensures that after a disruption, the patient is not only acknowledged but fully restored to the center of the conversation.

Example: Step 6—Reestablishing Structure and Presence

The sixth step is reestablishing structure and presence. Once the interaction is repaired, the healthcare provider resumes the encounter with clarity, maintaining the same standards of listening, explanation, and alignment.

The patient has resumed their narrative after being reinvited. The interruption has been repaired, and the interaction feels more balanced. Now the healthcare provider must guide the encounter forward without losing the restored connection. The healthcare provider maintains eye contact, posture steady and oriented toward the patient. A brief pause signals the transition.

Provider:
Thank you for explaining that. I want to make sure I understand everything clearly.

The tone is calm and organized.

Patient:
Okay.

Provider:
You mentioned the pressure started suddenly while you were at rest, and that's what concerned you most.

The healthcare provider reflects key elements, reinforcing understanding.

Patient:
Yes, exactly.

Provider:
I'm going to ask a few specific questions to get a complete picture.

The structure is reintroduced clearly. The healthcare provider proceeds with focused, measured questions.

Provider:
Since it started, has the pressure been constant, or does it come and go?

Patient:
It comes and goes.

Provider:
And when it happens, how long does it usually last?

Patient:
A few minutes.

The healthcare provider listens without interruption, maintaining presence. After several questions, the healthcare provider transitions again.

Provider:
I'm going to explain what I think may be happening and what we should do next.

The flow of the encounter is restored. The patient remains engaged, posture open. The earlier disruption is no longer influencing the interaction. The healthcare provider continues with clarity, pacing, and alignment.

What has been demonstrated is measurable:

- The healthcare provider reintroduced structure after the repair.
- Key information was summarized to confirm understanding.
- Focused questions resumed in an organized manner.
- Presence and attention were maintained throughout.
- The interaction returned to a clear, steady clinical flow.

This is reestablishing structure and presence. It ensures that once trust is repaired, the encounter continues with the same clarity, control, and patient-centered focus as if the disruption had not occurred. Repair does not weaken the interaction. When done well, it often strengthens it.

Patients do not expect perfection. They expect to be respected. When a healthcare provider recognizes a misstep and addresses it directly, it communicates humility, awareness, and professionalism. These qualities build trust more effectively than flawless execution.

Importantly, repair must be timely. Delayed acknowledgment loses relevance and impact. The closer the repair is to the moment of disruption, the more effective it becomes.

In many cases, the repaired interaction is what patients remember most, because it demonstrates something deeper than technical skill. It shows that the healthcare provider is not only present when things go smoothly, but also accountable when they do not. And in that accountability, trust is restored.

Chapter 27

The 10-Second Orientation Rule

Addressing the patient and the accompanying people

When a healthcare provider enters a room with a patient and accompanying people, there is a simple but powerful sequence that establishes respect, control, and clarity:

1. Pause, look up, and acknowledge the room before the chart

Even if the healthcare provider reviewed the chart outside, the first few seconds inside the room should belong to the people, not the paperwork. A brief pause, eye contact, and orientation to *who is present* signals awareness and respect.

2. Greet the patient first, then include others explicitly

The patient remains the center of care, but others in the room are not invisible. A healthcare provider might say to the patient, "Hi, I'm Dr.___, it's good to meet you," then turn to each person present with, "And you are?" This does two things:

- It acknowledges each person as a participant in the environment
- It allows the healthcare provider to understand roles (mother, partner, friend)

3. Clarify permission and roles early

This is a critical but often skipped step. The healthcare provider should confirm: "Are you comfortable discussing everything with them in the room?" This protects patient privacy and establishes boundaries in a respectful way. It also signals professionalism to everyone present.

4. Maintain shared eye contact, not tunnel vision

While most communication should be directed to the patient, occasional inclusion of others through eye contact or brief acknowledgment maintains a sense of inclusion without diluting the healthcare provider-patient relationship.

5. Avoid "chart-first behavior" once inside the room

Looking down and reading before engaging communicates hierarchy and detachment. It says, unintentionally, "the data matters more than the person."

Provider (*pauses at the door, looks up*):
Good morning.

Provider:
Hi, I'm Dr. Harris. It's nice to meet you.

Patient:
Nice to meet you, too.

Provider:
And you are?

Mother:
I'm her mother.

Provider:
Thank you for being here. And you?

Partner:
I'm her boyfriend.

Provider:
I appreciate you both coming to support her.

Provider:
Before we begin, are you comfortable discussing everything with them in the room?

Patient:
Yes, that's fine.

Provider:
Alright, thank you for letting me know.

Provider (*turns back to patient*):
What brought you in today?

Patient:
I've been having some chest discomfort.

Provider:
I'm glad you came in. We'll go through this carefully.

Provider *(brief eye contact with others)*:
And feel free to add anything you think is important.

Mother:
She mentioned it started a few days ago.

Provider:
Thank you, that's helpful.

Provider (returns focus to patient):
Can you describe what it feels like?

Patient:
It's more of a pressure than pain.

Provider:
When did you first notice it?

Patient:
About three days ago.

Provider:
Has anything made it better or worse?

Patient:
It gets worse when I walk.

Provider (nods, maintains eye contact):
That's important to note.

Provider (brief glance to partner):
Have you noticed anything else?

Partner:
She's been more tired than usual.

Provider:
Thank you. That adds useful context.

Provider (back to patient):
We'll make sure we look at this from every angle.

Provider:
I'm going to ask a few more questions, then we'll discuss next steps together.

Patient:
Okay.

Provider:
You're in the right place. Let's take this step by step.

What Is Considered Standard Etiquette Today

In reality, what you experienced is unfortunately common. Many healthcare providers are trained in efficiency-driven environments where:

- The chart is prioritized immediately upon entry
- The patient is addressed, but others are ignored unless they speak
- Consent for others being present is assumed rather than confirmed
- Time pressure overrides relational awareness

So, while the behavior you saw is common, it is not ideal, and increasingly, it is being recognized as a deficiency in modern care.

The Room Is a System, Not Just a Patient

When a healthcare provider ignores others present:

- They miss context (family dynamics, support systems, concerns)
- They reduce trust among those influencing the patient's care
- They unintentionally create emotional distance at the very start of the visit

And importantly, patients often *experience care through the lens of those around them*. If a mother or partner feels dismissed, that perception feeds back into the patient's sense of care.

The 10-Second Orientation Rule

Within the first 10 seconds of entering the room, the healthcare provider should:

1. Make eye contact with the patient
2. Acknowledge every person present
3. Identify roles
4. Confirm consent for shared discussion

This takes less than half a minute, yet it transforms the entire encounter.

Conclusion: The Provider Patients Never Forget

What has been presented is not just about politeness. It is about presence, awareness, and intentional structure in human interaction, which is often missing in healthcare training. It is precisely these small, repeatable behaviors that define the quality of care people remember.

Patients do not remember every detail of their care. They do not recall every question asked, every term used, or every step of the examination. What they remember is how they were treated in the moments that mattered most. They remember the healthcare provider who looked at them before looking at the chart. The one who allowed them to speak without interruption. The one who reflected their words back with clarity, showing true understanding. The one who explained things in a way that reduced fear instead of increasing it. The one who stayed steady in moments of uncertainty. The one who paused, noticed, and repaired when something felt off.

These are not extraordinary acts. They are consistent, repeatable behaviors. What distinguishes the provider patients never forget is not perfection. It is presence. It is the ability to enter a room with awareness. To listen without rushing. To communicate with clarity and intention. To recognize when something has shifted and to restore it.

These skills do not require more time. They require attention. And over time, they become identity. The healthcare provider who practices this way does not think of these actions as techniques. They become natural, embedded in every interaction, across every setting. Patients sense this immediately. It is reflected not in what is said about the healthcare provider, but in how patients feel when they leave. They feel seen. They feel heard. They feel understood. They feel supported. That is what they remember.

In the end, medicine is not only defined by outcomes, but by experience. And experience is shaped in moments—small, precise, and entirely within the healthcare provider's control. The provider patients never forget is the one who understands that care begins before the first word is spoken, continues through every interaction, and remains long after the visit has ended.

Chapter 28

The Waiting Room Problem

Why Patients Wait… And What It Communicates

Modern medicine does not intentionally set out to make patients wait. Yet the experience of waiting, often for extended periods, has become one of the most common and frustrating aspects of healthcare. Patients notice it immediately. They remember it. And more importantly, they interpret it.

From the healthcare provider's perspective, overbooking is rarely about disregard. It is driven by competing demands: unpredictable visit lengths, urgent add-ons, administrative burdens, and the pressure to maintain financial viability. A schedule that appears reasonable on paper often collapses under the weight of real-world variability. One complex patient can delay an entire morning. Multiply that across a day, and delays become inevitable.

But from the patient's perspective, the meaning is very different. Waiting is not experienced as a scheduling issue. It is experienced as a signal. It can feel like:

- *My time is less valuable*
- *I am not a priority*
- *No one is aware of me sitting here*

And when that perception forms, it begins shaping the relationship before the healthcare provider even enters the room.

This is where awareness becomes critical. Most healthcare providers do recognize that delays occur. What is often underestimated is the emotional impact of unacknowledged waiting. Silence in the waiting room creates interpretation. And interpretation, in the absence of communication, often becomes negative.

Waiting Room Interaction: When Time Becomes Emotion

Patient *(approaching the front desk, visibly frustrated)*:
Excuse me… I've been waiting for over 45 minutes. I had a 2:15 appointment. It's now 3:00.
What's going on?

Receptionist (typing, without looking up immediately):
We're running a little behind today.

Patient:
A little behind? This isn't a little behind. This is almost an hour.

Receptionist (still neutral tone):
The doctor is with patients. It happens sometimes.

Patient (voice tightening):
I understand that. But no one said anything. I've just been sitting there with no update. Am I even checked in?

Receptionist (glances briefly):
Yes, you're checked in.

Patient:
Then why didn't anyone tell me there was a delay?

Receptionist (slight pause):
We've been busy.

Patient (now clearly irritated):
I rearranged my entire afternoon to be here on time. If I showed up 45 minutes late, would I still be seen?

Receptionist (defensive tone):
That's different.

Patient:
No, it's not. My time matters too.

(There is a pause. The receptionist softens slightly.)

Receptionist:
I understand. The doctor had a complicated case earlier, and it backed things up. You should be next.

Patient (exhales, still frustrated but calmer):
That's all I needed to hear. Just… someone telling me what's going on.

(A moment of silence. The emotional tone shifts slightly.)

Patient (quieter):
It just feels like no one notices we're sitting out there.

Receptionist (more attentive now):
I'm sorry. I should have let you know sooner.

What This Interaction Reveals

The frustration was not caused solely by the delay. It was shaped by:

- Lack of acknowledgment
- Lack of communication
- Perception of being overlooked

When the receptionist finally provided a simple explanation, the patient's tone changed immediately. Not because the wait was shorter, but because the experience was finally recognized.

Alternative Interaction (Same Situation, Different Approach)

Receptionist (proactively, as patient approaches):
Hi, I just wanted to let you know the doctor is running about 30–40 minutes behind due to a complicated case. I'm really sorry for the delay.

Patient (still concerned, but calmer):
Okay… thank you for letting me know.

Receptionist:
If you need to step out or reschedule, I can help with that. Otherwise, we'll get you in as soon as possible.

Patient:
No, I'll wait. I appreciate you telling me.

Contrast

In both scenarios, the delay is identical, but the experience is not because in the second interaction:

- The patient is acknowledged
- The delay is explained
- The patient is given a sense of control

Closing Reflection

The waiting room is not silent. It is filled with interpretation. Every interaction, or lack of one, shapes the relationship before the healthcare provider ever enters the room. The issue, therefore, is not simply overbooking. It is the *absence of transparency and acknowledgment.*

A patient who waits 30 minutes with no explanation feels dismissed. A patient who waits the same 30 minutes but is informed, updated, and acknowledged experiences something entirely different.

The solution does not require perfection in scheduling. That is unrealistic. It requires intentional communication. Simple changes can transform the experience:

- Acknowledging delays early

- Providing realistic time expectations
- Offering patients choices when delays become significant
- Beginning the encounter with recognition: *"I know you've been waiting, and I appreciate your patience."*

These moments are small, but their impact is disproportionate because the waiting room is not just a physical space; it is the first test of the relationship. Before any diagnosis is made, before any treatment is discussed, the patient is already forming conclusions about respect, value, and attentiveness. And those conclusions matter.

Key Insight

Overbooking may be a system necessity. Overbooking often feels like a disregard for patients' time, but in reality, it is usually a response to the **unpredictable nature of medical care** rather than a deliberate choice to inconvenience.

In clinical practice, no two visits are truly the same. A scheduled 15-minute appointment may become 30 minutes if a patient presents with unexpected symptoms, emotional distress, or complex medical issues. Healthcare providers are not simply moving through a checklist. They are responding in real time to human variability, and that variability cannot be perfectly predicted when the schedule is created.

In addition, healthcare systems operate under constant pressure to **increase access.** There are always more patients needing care than there are available appointment slots. Overbooking becomes a way to reduce long wait times for appointments, accommodate urgent cases, and ensure that patients are not turned away when they need to be seen.

There is also a practical reality that not all patients arrive on time or attend their appointments. Without some degree of overbooking, gaps would appear in the schedule, reducing efficiency and limiting how many patients can be cared for in a day. In that sense, overbooking is used to **balance unpredictability with access.**

However, while overbooking may be a system necessity, its impact is felt at the individual level. Patients do not experience it as a strategy. They experience it as waiting. This is where the distinction becomes critical. The issue is not the existence of overbooking itself. The issue is how its consequences are managed.

When delays are acknowledged, explained, and handled with transparency, patients are far more understanding. When they are left waiting without communication, the same system necessity becomes a relational failure.

Overbooking may help the system function. But without awareness and communication, it can quietly undermine the very relationships on which healthcare depends. A healthcare provider who consistently runs behind is not dealing with an occasional disruption. They are dealing with a predictable pattern, and predictable patterns can be redesigned.

Reframing the Problem

The goal is not to eliminate all delays. That is unrealistic. The goal is to eliminate the emotional damage caused by those delays. Patients will tolerate waiting. They will not tolerate feeling ignored. An office that has a chronic scheduling problem hinders patient relationships.

1. Acknowledge that this is a system issue, not a patient issue

If delays happen daily, the problem is not "a busy day." It is a structural scheduling problem. This requires:

- Reviewing average visit lengths honestly
- Identifying which visit types consistently run over
- Adjusting scheduling templates accordingly

Many offices schedule based on ideal time. They should schedule based on real time.

2. Build buffer into the schedule

Back-to-back scheduling with no margin guarantees delays. Instead:

- Add intentional buffer slots every 2–3 patients
- Use those buffers to absorb overruns

This alone can dramatically reduce cascading delays throughout the day

3. Use tiered appointment lengths

Not all visits should be treated equally.
Examples:

- Routine follow-up → shorter
- New patient or complex issues → longer
- Emotional or multi-issue visits → extended slots

When everything is scheduled the same, everything runs late.

4. Communicate delays proactively

This is one of the most powerful and underused tools. The office should:

- Inform patients at check-in if delays exist
- Provide realistic expectations ("about 30 minutes behind")
- Offer options when delays are significant

Patients don't expect perfection. They expect awareness.

5. Train front desk staff to manage emotion, not just flow

Front desk staff are not just administrative. They are the emotional gatekeepers of the experience. They should be trained to:

- Make eye contact
- Acknowledge wait times sincerely
- Avoid dismissive language like, "We're busy."
- Use validating language:
    - "I understand this is frustrating."
    - "Thank you for your patience."

This alone can change the tone of the entire visit.

6. Reset the relationship when entering the room

The healthcare provider must recognize that the patient has already had an experience before the encounter begins. A simple statement matters: "I know you've been waiting, and I appreciate your patience." This does three things:

- Acknowledges reality
- Demonstrates awareness
- Rebuilds respect

Without this, the patient may remain emotionally distant throughout the visit.

7. Use technology to improve transparency

Simple systems can help:

- Text updates for delays
- Digital check-in with time estimates
- Notifications allowing patients to step out briefly

These tools restore a sense of control.

8. Measure and monitor wait times

What is not measured is not improved. Track:

- Average wait times
- Peak delay periods
- Patient feedback related to waiting

Patterns will emerge. Solutions become clearer.

9. Consider cultural change within the office

If long waits are accepted as "just how it is," nothing will improve. The culture should shift to:

- Respect for patient time as a core value
- Awareness that waiting affects relationships
- Shared responsibility across the team

10. Understand the True Cost

Long waits do more than frustrate patients. They lead to:

- Decreased satisfaction
- Reduced trust
- Lower adherence to care
- Negative word-of-mouth

In other words, they directly impact outcomes and reputation.

Closing Insight

A healthcare provider who consistently runs behind is not simply managing time; they are managing perception, respect, and trust. Overbooking may be necessary, but unmanaged waiting is optional. When addressed thoughtfully, even a delayed schedule can still produce a strong, respectful, and trusting relationship.

Chapter 29

Setting the Patient's Expectations — The Process Explained

Often, when patients come into the office with a health concern, their expectations are understandably high. They are seeking relief, clarity, and, in many cases, a quick resolution to their problem. Pain, discomfort, and uncertainty naturally create a desire for immediate answers and rapid improvement.

However, a gap often exists between what the patient expects and what the provider believes is the realistic course of healing. When this gap is not addressed through clear communication, expectations can become misaligned. Patients may anticipate rapid results, while the actual process of diagnosis, treatment, and recovery may require time, patience, and ongoing evaluation.

Without proper explanation, this disconnect can lead to frustration. Patients may begin to feel that their concerns are not being resolved effectively and, in some cases, question the provider's competence. What is often a normal and appropriate medical process can instead be perceived as inadequate care.

A simple, thoughtful explanation of the healing process can significantly improve this dynamic. When providers take the time to outline what to expect, including timelines, possible outcomes, and uncertainties, patients are better equipped to align their expectations with reality. This shared understanding strengthens trust, reduces frustration, and ultimately supports a more effective and collaborative relationship.

In that explanation, the provider must also communicate that treatment plans are not always fixed. As care progresses, adjustments may be necessary, particularly when results are not meeting expectations. This is not a failure of care, but rather a reflection of the body's complexity and the individualized nature of healing.

It is important for patients to understand that no single approach guarantees a predictable outcome. What works effectively for one individual may not produce the same results for another. For this reason, part of setting expectations involves preparing the patient for the possibility of redirection. Treatment may need to be refined, adjusted, or even changed in order to better align with the patient's response and the underlying condition.

Patients should also be made aware that alternative methods may sometimes be required to achieve the most comprehensive results. This is one of the reasons why the process of healing takes both time and patience. There is rarely a true "quick fix." Instead, progress unfolds through careful observation, measured interventions, and ongoing reassessment.

Follow-up visits play a critical role in this process. They allow the provider to evaluate outcomes using both subjective feedback from the patient and objective clinical findings. These reassessments guide decision-making, ensuring that treatment remains aligned with the patient's needs and continues to move toward the best possible outcome.

Dialogue 1: The Urgent Expectation

Patient:
Doctor, I've had this back pain for two weeks now. I need something that fixes it quickly. I can't keep living like this.

Provider:
I understand how disruptive that kind of pain can be. When something affects your daily life, it's natural to want immediate relief. Let's talk about what's going on and what we can realistically expect moving forward.

Patient:
So you can fix it today?

Provider:
We can absolutely start helping you today, but healing often doesn't happen instantly. Back pain, especially when it develops over time, usually improves in stages. Our goal is to reduce your pain, restore function, and prevent it from returning, but that process may take some time.

Patient:
That's frustrating. I was hoping for something faster.

Provider:
That makes sense. Many people feel that way. What's important is that we approach this in a way that actually works long term. Sometimes quick fixes can mask the issue without truly resolving it.

Patient:
So what happens next?

Provider:
We'll begin with a treatment plan based on what I'm seeing today. As we move forward, we'll monitor how your body responds. If something isn't giving us the results we expect, we'll adjust. That's a normal part of care, not a setback.

Patient:
So it's more of a process?

Provider:
Exactly. And I'll guide you through each step, so you know what to expect. That way, nothing feels uncertain or out of control.

Dialogue 2: The Doubtful Patient

Patient:
I've already tried treatment before, and it didn't work. I don't want to waste time again.

Provider:
I hear that. When something doesn't work, it can be discouraging and even make you question whether anything will help.

Patient:
Exactly. That's why I'm skeptical.

Provider:
That's completely reasonable. What's important to understand is that not all treatments work the same for every person. The body is complex, and sometimes it takes adjusting our approach to find what truly works for you.

Patient:
So you're saying this might not work either?

Provider:
What I'm saying is that we'll start with a plan based on your condition and your history. If your response isn't what we expect, we won't stay stuck. We'll reassess and modify the approach. That flexibility is part of good care.

Patient:
So it's not just one plan and that's it?

Provider:
Exactly. Think of it as a guided process rather than a single attempt. We evaluate both how you feel and what we observe clinically. That combination helps us move in the right direction.

Patient:
That actually makes more sense than what I've experienced before.

Provider:
And I'll make sure you understand each step along the way. That way, we're working together, not just trying things blindly.

Dialogue 3: The Impatient Follow-Up

Patient:
I came last week, and I don't feel that much better. Is the treatment even working?

Provider:
I appreciate you bringing that up. It's important that we talk about how you're feeling and what you're noticing.

Patient:
I thought I'd feel a lot better by now.

Provider:
That's a very common expectation. Early in treatment, improvements can sometimes be gradual rather than immediate. What we look for at this stage is whether there are small changes, even if they're not dramatic yet.

Patient:
I guess it's a little less intense but not gone.

Provider:
That's actually meaningful progress. It tells us your body is responding, even if it's not as quickly as you hoped.

Patient:
So we just keep doing the same thing?

Provider:
Not necessarily. This is where follow-up visits are important. We use what you're experiencing, along with what I'm seeing clinically, to decide whether to continue, adjust, or refine the plan.

Patient:
So you're constantly evaluating it?

Provider:
Exactly. Treatment is dynamic. If needed, we'll shift direction to better match your response. That's how we move toward the best outcome.

Patient:
That makes me feel better about coming back.

Provider:
Good. These visits are not just routine; they're essential to making sure we're on the right path.

Dialogue 4: The Educated Alignment

Patient:
I just want to understand what this process is going to look like. I don't want surprises.

Provider:
That's a very helpful approach, and I'm glad you said that. Let me walk you through what you can expect.

Patient:
Please.

Provider:
First, we begin with an initial treatment based on your condition. From there, we observe how your body responds. Healing is not always linear, so we may see improvement, plateaus, or even the need to adjust direction.

Patient:
So it's not a straight line to getting better?

Provider:
Exactly. And that's normal. Part of setting expectations is understanding that we may need to modify treatment if results aren't progressing as we'd like.

Patient:
Does that mean trying completely different methods?

Provider:
Sometimes, yes. There are often multiple ways to approach a condition. If one method doesn't provide the desired outcome, we explore alternatives to find what works best for you.

Patient:
And that's why it takes time?

Provider:
Yes. Effective care is about precision, not speed. There's rarely a true quick fix, especially for complex conditions. What matters is that we're consistently moving in the right direction.

Patient:
And the follow-ups are to track that?

Provider:
Exactly. We use both your experience, what you feel, and objective findings, what we can measure, to guide decisions. That way, your care remains aligned with your needs at every stage.

Patient:
I feel much more comfortable knowing that.

Provider:
That understanding is one of the most important parts of the process. It allows us to work together with clarity and trust.

Conclusion

The Healthcare Provider Patients Never Forget

Patients do not remember every detail of their care. They do not recall every question asked, every term used, or every step of the examination. What they remember is how they were treated in the moments that mattered most.

They remember the healthcare provider who looked at them before looking at the chart. The one who allowed them to speak without interruption. The one who reflected their words back with clarity, showing true understanding. The one who explained things in a way that reduced fear instead of increasing it. The one who stayed steady in moments of uncertainty. The one who paused, noticed, and repaired when something felt off. These are not extraordinary acts. They are consistent, repeatable behaviors.

What distinguishes the healthcare provider patients never forget is not perfection. It is presence. It is the ability to enter a room with awareness. To listen without rushing. To communicate with clarity and intention. To recognize when something has shifted and to restore it. These skills do not require more time. They require attention and over time, they become identity.

The healthcare provider who practices this way does not think of these actions as techniques. They become natural, embedded in every interaction, across every setting. Patients sense this immediately. It is reflected not in what is said about the healthcare provider, but in how patients feel when they leave: they feel seen, they feel heard, they feel understood, they feel supported. That is what they remember.

In the end, medicine is not only defined by outcomes, but by experience. And experience is shaped in moments — small, precise, and entirely within the healthcare provider's control. The healthcare provider patients never forget is the one who understands that care begins before the first word is spoken, continues through every interaction, and remains long after the visit has ended.

Acknowledgments

This book would not exist without the countless patients, healthcare professionals, educators, colleagues, and students whose experiences helped shape the ideas within these pages.

First and foremost, I want to acknowledge the patients who entrusted healthcare providers with their fears, vulnerabilities, questions, and hopes during some of the most uncertain moments of their lives. Every interaction between a patient and provider carries lessons that extend far beyond medicine itself. The strength, honesty, and humanity shown by patients continue to remind us why compassionate care matters.

I also extend my deepest appreciation to the physicians, nurses, physician assistants, nurse practitioners, medical assistants, caregivers, administrators, and support staff who dedicate themselves daily to the service of others. Healthcare is often practiced under extraordinary pressure, yet so many professionals continue to offer comfort, reassurance, and dignity even in the most demanding environments. Your work inspires this book.

To medical educators and mentors who recognize that communication, emotional awareness, and relationship-building deserve equal importance alongside clinical training—thank you for helping shape a more human-centered future in medicine.

I am especially grateful to the many colleagues and learners who shared their experiences openly, allowing important conversations about trust, communication, burnout, empathy, and patient care to take place honestly and thoughtfully. Those discussions reinforced the belief that relational skills are not secondary in healthcare—they are foundational.

Appendix A

Part I — First Impressions and Trust

Questions 1–20

1. Why are first impressions so influential in medicine?

A. They determine billing accuracy.

B. They shape patient trust and emotional safety.

C. They shorten every appointment.

D. They eliminate patient anxiety.

2. How quickly do patients begin evaluating healthcare providers?

A. After receiving treatment recommendations.

B. After laboratory results are reviewed.

C. Within the first few seconds of interaction.

D. Only after the physical examination.

3. What silent question are patients often asking during the first interaction?

A. "How expensive will this visit be?"

B. "Can I trust this person with my care?"

C. "Will this appointment be short?"

D. "Does this provider prefer technology?"

4. Why does eye contact matter in clinical encounters?

A. It improves computer efficiency.

B. It communicates attentiveness and presence.

C. It reduces the need for explanation.

D. It shortens documentation time.

5. How can posture influence patient trust?

A. Patients unconsciously interpret body language emotionally.

B. Posture increases prescription compliance automatically.

C. Posture removes uncertainty completely.

D. Posture eliminates emotional reactions.

6. Why do patients interpret rushed behavior negatively?

A. It signals emotional unavailability or lack of time.

B. It demonstrates leadership and authority.

C. It improves confidence immediately.

D. It increases emotional safety.

7. What emotional signals does calmness communicate?

A. Emotional instability.

B. Indifference toward patients.

C. Steadiness, control, and reassurance.

D. Uncertainty and hesitation.

8. How does a provider's tone affect patient perception?

A. Tone shapes emotional interpretation of communication.

B. Tone has little effect on patients.

C. Tone replaces medical skill.

D. Tone prevents difficult conversations.

9. Why is psychological safety important during patient interactions?

A. It prevents all emotional reactions.

B. It helps patients feel secure enough to communicate openly.

C. It shortens medical visits automatically.

D. It removes diagnostic uncertainty completely.

10. How can body orientation affect communication?

A. Patients interpret body positioning emotionally.

B. Body orientation improves billing accuracy.

C. Body orientation eliminates anxiety completely.

D. Body orientation prevents patient questions.

11. Why does sitting down often improve patient trust?

A. It shortens the appointment.

B. It creates emotional equality and attentiveness.

C. It prevents difficult emotions.

D. It reduces the need for explanation.

12. What role does attentiveness play in relationship-building?

A. Patients associate attentiveness with genuine caring.

B. Attentiveness weakens professionalism.

C. Attentiveness increases emotional distance.

D. Attentiveness removes uncertainty instantly.

13. How can distractions damage rapport?

A. Patients may feel emotionally unimportant or unheard.

B. Distractions improve trust automatically.

C. Distractions strengthen communication.

D. Distractions reduce emotional sensitivity.

14. Why is presence more important than perfection?

A. Patients emotionally remember how providers made them feel.

B. Perfection weakens trust.

C. Presence eliminates medical mistakes.

D. Presence replaces competence.

15. How do patients interpret interruptions?

A. As evidence of deep listening.

B. As signs that they are being rushed or dismissed.

C. As emotional reassurance.

D. As proof of efficiency only.

16. What is the relationship between listening and trust?

A. Listening helps patients feel understood and respected.

B. Listening weakens efficiency.

C. Listening replaces diagnosis.

D. Listening prevents emotional discussions.

17. Why is respect communicated nonverbally?

A. Patients interpret behavior emotionally before intellectually.

B. Respect depends only on spoken words.

C. Nonverbal behavior has little influence.

D. Respect is unrelated to communication.

18. How can first impressions influence long-term outcomes?

A. They shape trust, openness, and treatment cooperation.

B. They only affect waiting room satisfaction.

C. They replace clinical skill.

D. They eliminate patient fear permanently.

19. Why do patients remember interactions more than medical details?

A. Emotional experiences are deeply remembered.

B. Patients ignore all medical information.

C. Technical knowledge is emotionally irrelevant.

D. Emotions weaken memory completely.

20. How does emotional awareness improve patient care?

A. It helps providers recognize and respond to emotional needs.

B. It replaces clinical competence.

C. It eliminates uncertainty completely.

D. It prevents all difficult conversations.

Part II — Communication Skills

Questions 21–40

21. Why is communication considered a clinical skill?

A. Communication replaces diagnosis.

B. Communication directly affects trust, understanding, and outcomes.

C. Communication only improves office efficiency.

D. Communication prevents all medical errors.

22. How does clear communication reduce patient anxiety?

A. It eliminates all uncertainty immediately.

B. It helps patients understand what is happening and what comes next.

C. It removes emotional reactions completely.

D. It prevents difficult conversations.

23. Why must healthcare providers avoid overly technical language?

A. Patients may feel confused, overwhelmed, or disconnected.

B. Technical language weakens medical knowledge.

C. Patients prefer emotional conversations only.

D. Technical language prevents diagnosis.

24. What happens when patients feel confused during explanations?

A. Trust and confidence may weaken.

B. Anxiety disappears immediately.

C. Patients feel emotionally reassured.

D. Communication improves automatically.

25. Why should providers check for understanding?

A. Patients always understand explanations immediately.

B. Confirming understanding improves clarity and reduces confusion.

C. Checking understanding weakens authority.

D. It prevents emotional conversations.

26. What is the danger of vague communication?

A. Patients may feel unsupported and uncertain.

B. Vagueness increases emotional safety.

C. Vague communication strengthens trust automatically.

D. Vagueness removes patient anxiety.

27. Why is clarity associated with competence?

A. Organized explanations communicate confidence and understanding.

B. Clarity weakens professionalism.

C. Patients dislike clear explanations.

D. Confusion improves trust.

28. How does tone affect difficult conversations?

A. Tone shapes emotional interpretation and comfort.

B. Tone is unrelated to patient emotions.

C. Tone replaces honesty.

D. Tone prevents emotional reactions.

29. Why is pacing important during communication?

A. Patients need time to emotionally and mentally process information.

B. Fast pacing always improves trust.

C. Slow pacing prevents honesty.

D. Pacing eliminates anxiety completely.

30. How can pauses improve patient interactions?

A. Pauses create emotional and cognitive processing space.

B. Pauses weaken communication.

C. Pauses eliminate emotional reactions.

D. Pauses replace empathy.

31. Why must providers avoid appearing rushed?

A. Patients may interpret rushing as emotional unavailability.

B. Rushing strengthens connection.

C. Rushed behavior improves reassurance.

D. Rushing removes patient fear.

32. What is the impact of dismissive language?

A. Patients may feel invalidated or emotionally unimportant.

B. Dismissive language strengthens trust.

C. Dismissive language improves emotional safety.

D. Dismissive language reduces confusion automatically.

33. Why should communication be individualized?

A. Every patient processes information and emotion differently.

B. All patients communicate the same way.

C. Individualized communication weakens efficiency.

D. Communication style has little importance.

34. How can empathy improve patient cooperation?

A. Patients are more likely to trust and follow guidance when they feel understood.

B. Empathy replaces treatment plans.

C. Empathy prevents difficult conversations.

D. Empathy eliminates anxiety permanently.

35. Why are reflective statements effective?

A. They demonstrate listening and emotional understanding.

B. They replace diagnosis.

C. They shorten appointments automatically.

D. They eliminate uncertainty.

36. How can providers communicate uncertainty without weakening trust?

A. By explaining what is known and outlining clear next steps.

B. By avoiding difficult discussions.

C. By pretending certainty exists.

D. By minimizing patient concerns.

37. Why should providers explain "next steps"?

A. Patients feel more emotionally grounded when they understand the process.

B. Explanations increase confusion.

C. Patients prefer uncertainty.

D. Next steps are emotionally unimportant.

38. What role does reassurance play in medicine?

A. Reassurance helps reduce emotional distress when combined with honesty and clarity.

B. Reassurance replaces treatment.

C. Reassurance eliminates fear permanently.

D. Reassurance prevents all grief.

39. How can providers avoid minimizing patient fears?

A. By validating emotional concerns respectfully.

B. By dismissing emotional reactions quickly.

C. By avoiding difficult emotions.

D. By focusing only on technical information.

40. Why do patients value honesty?

A. Trust depends on truthful and transparent communication.

B. Honesty weakens reassurance.

C. Patients prefer uncertainty and confusion.

D. Emotional comfort matters more than truth.

Part III — Competence and Connection

Questions 41–60

41. Why do patients merge competence and connection into one perception?

A. Patients separate emotions completely from medical care.

B. Patients experience competence and human connection together.

C. Patients only focus on technical skill.

D. Patients ignore emotional interactions.

42. How can connection strengthen trust in competence?

A. Emotional connection helps patients feel safer accepting guidance.

B. Connection replaces clinical knowledge.

C. Connection prevents uncertainty completely.

D. Connection eliminates emotional reactions.

43. Why is warmth alone insufficient in healthcare?

A. Patients also need clarity, direction, and leadership.

B. Warmth weakens professionalism.

C. Warmth prevents trust.

D. Warmth replaces competence entirely.

44. What happens when competence feels inaccessible?

A. Patients may feel confused or emotionally disconnected.

B. Trust automatically increases.

C. Emotional safety improves completely.

D. Patients stop asking questions.

45. Why do patients need leadership during uncertainty?

A. Leadership provides emotional stability and direction.

B. Leadership removes all fear instantly.

C. Leadership replaces empathy.

D. Leadership avoids difficult conversations.

46. How can structure reduce patient anxiety?

A. Structure helps patients understand what to expect next.

B. Structure prevents emotions completely.

C. Structure eliminates uncertainty permanently.

D. Structure weakens communication.

47. Why does confidence matter in healthcare communication?

A. Calm confidence reassures vulnerable patients.

B. Confidence eliminates medical errors completely.

C. Confidence replaces emotional awareness.

D. Confidence prevents grief.

48. How is quiet confidence different from arrogance?

A. Quiet confidence combines calmness with humility and clarity.

B. Quiet confidence avoids communication.

C. Quiet confidence dominates patients emotionally.

D. Quiet confidence eliminates empathy.

49. Why is accessibility important in communication?

A. Patients need information explained in understandable ways.

B. Accessibility weakens professionalism.

C. Patients prefer confusion.

D. Accessibility prevents emotional reactions.

50. How can competence appear weakened by poor delivery?

A. Patients may interpret unclear communication as uncertainty.

B. Poor delivery strengthens trust automatically.

C. Communication style has no effect on perception.

D. Competence removes emotional interpretation.

51. Why does emotional intelligence strengthen clinical care?

A. Emotional awareness improves trust, understanding, and cooperation.

B. Emotional intelligence replaces diagnosis.

C. Emotional intelligence weakens leadership.

D. Emotional intelligence prevents difficult emotions.

52. What happens when connection feels hollow?

A. Patients may feel emotionally supported but not guided.

B. Trust becomes automatically stronger.

C. Emotional safety increases completely.

D. Patients stop needing reassurance.

53. Why must providers guide as well as support?

A. Patients need both compassion and direction.

B. Guidance weakens emotional safety.

C. Support replaces leadership.

D. Guidance eliminates emotional reactions.

54. How can uncertainty damage trust if poorly communicated?

A. Patients may feel abandoned or unsupported.

B. Uncertainty always improves reassurance.

C. Patients prefer vague explanations.

D. Emotional reactions disappear during uncertainty.

55. Why are patients highly sensitive to emotional signals?

A. Vulnerability increases emotional awareness and perception.

B. Emotional signals are medically irrelevant.

C. Patients ignore provider behavior.

D. Emotions weaken trust formation.

56. How does attentiveness influence perceived expertise?

A. Patients associate careful listening with thoroughness and competence.

B. Attentiveness weakens professionalism.

C. Patients dislike attentive providers.

D. Expertise is unrelated to communication.

57. Why should providers explain their reasoning?

A. Transparency strengthens understanding and trust.

B. Patients prefer unexplained decisions.

C. Explanations weaken authority.

D. Reasoning increases confusion automatically.

58. What role does leadership play in medicine?

A. Leadership helps patients feel guided through uncertainty.

B. Leadership replaces empathy entirely.

C. Leadership avoids emotional conversations.

D. Leadership eliminates difficult decisions.

59. Why do patients seek both safety and direction?

A. Patients need emotional reassurance and clear guidance simultaneously.

B. Patients only value emotional comfort.

C. Direction weakens trust.

D. Safety replaces communication.

60. How can connection stabilize difficult encounters?

A. Human connection reduces fear, isolation, and emotional distress.

B. Connection eliminates grief permanently.

C. Connection removes the need for honesty.

D. Difficult encounters should avoid emotional support.

Part IV — Emotional Awareness

Questions 61–80

61. Why must healthcare providers recognize patient fear?

A. Fear affects emotional stability and communication.

B. Fear has no influence on patient behavior.

C. Fear improves understanding automatically.

D. Fear eliminates emotional reactions.

62. How does anxiety affect patient understanding?

A. Anxiety can reduce concentration and information retention.

B. Anxiety improves memory perfectly.

C. Anxiety removes emotional sensitivity.

D. Anxiety prevents fear entirely.

63. Why do emotions influence patient behavior?

A. Emotions affect trust, decision-making, and cooperation.

B. Emotions are unrelated to healthcare.

C. Emotions weaken all communication.

D. Emotions only affect families, not patients.

64. How can providers de-escalate emotional situations?

A. By remaining calm, respectful, and emotionally grounded.

B. By becoming defensive immediately.

C. By ignoring emotional reactions.

D. By speaking more aggressively.

65. Why is validation important?

A. Validation helps patients feel emotionally understood.

B. Validation weakens professionalism.

C. Validation prevents all emotional reactions.

D. Validation replaces diagnosis.

66. What is emotional regulation?

A. The ability to manage emotions while remaining present and professional.

B. The elimination of all emotional reactions.

C. Avoiding difficult conversations completely.

D. Ignoring emotional distress.

67. Why should providers avoid defensiveness?

A. Defensiveness can intensify emotional tension and weaken trust.

B. Defensiveness improves leadership automatically.

C. Defensiveness reduces anxiety immediately.

D. Defensiveness strengthens empathy.

68. How can emotional detachment harm care?

A. Patients may feel emotionally abandoned or uncared for.

B. Emotional detachment improves trust.

C. Emotional detachment eliminates grief.

D. Emotional detachment strengthens communication.

69. What is the difference between detachment and emotional control?

A. Emotional control remains compassionate while detachment withdraws emotionally.

B. Both are identical concepts.

C. Emotional control avoids empathy.

D. Detachment improves emotional connection.

70. Why is empathy essential in difficult conversations?

A. Empathy helps patients feel emotionally supported during vulnerability.

B. Empathy weakens professionalism.

C. Empathy prevents honesty.

D. Empathy eliminates grief completely.

71. How can emotional awareness improve outcomes?

A. Emotional awareness strengthens communication and cooperation.

B. Emotional awareness replaces treatment plans.

C. Emotional awareness weakens leadership.

D. Emotional awareness prevents uncertainty.

72. Why must providers remain calm under pressure?

A. Emotional steadiness reassures patients during stressful moments.

B. Calmness removes all emotional reactions.

C. Calmness replaces competence.

D. Calmness eliminates difficult conversations.

73. How does emotional presence build trust?

A. Patients feel less alone and more emotionally supported.

B. Emotional presence weakens authority.

C. Emotional presence prevents sadness entirely.

D. Emotional presence replaces treatment.

74. Why should providers acknowledge fear directly?

A. Recognition of fear helps patients feel emotionally understood.

B. Fear should always be ignored.

C. Acknowledging fear weakens reassurance.

D. Fear is emotionally unimportant.

75. What happens when patients feel emotionally dismissed?

A. Trust and openness may decrease significantly.

B. Patients become more cooperative automatically.

C. Emotional safety improves immediately.

D. Communication becomes easier.

76. Why is patience critical in healthcare?

A. Patients process emotions and information at different speeds.

B. Patience weakens efficiency completely.

C. Patience removes professionalism.

D. Patience eliminates uncertainty instantly.

77. How can providers reduce feelings of helplessness?

A. By offering clarity, guidance, and emotional support.

B. By avoiding difficult conversations.

C. By minimizing emotional concerns.

D. By focusing only on technical information.

78. Why does understanding patient emotion matter clinically?

A. Emotions influence behavior, trust, and treatment adherence.

B. Emotions are unrelated to healthcare outcomes.

C. Understanding emotion weakens competence.

D. Emotional awareness prevents diagnosis.

79. How can compassion improve communication?

A. Compassion strengthens emotional connection and trust.

B. Compassion replaces leadership.

C. Compassion weakens professionalism.

D. Compassion removes all anxiety permanently.

80. Why is emotional stability reassuring to patients?

A. Calm emotional presence creates feelings of safety and confidence.

B. Emotional stability prevents grief completely.

C. Emotional stability replaces treatment plans.

D. Emotional stability weakens emotional awareness.

Part V — Listening Skills

Questions 81–100

81. Why is listening considered diagnostic?

A. Listening reveals emotional and clinical information important for care.

B. Listening replaces physical examinations completely.

C. Listening weakens efficiency.

D. Listening prevents patient emotions.

82. How does interruption affect patient trust?

A. Patients may feel dismissed or emotionally unimportant.

B. Interruptions improve emotional safety automatically.

C. Interruptions strengthen communication.

D. Interruptions reduce anxiety immediately.

83. Why should providers allow patients to tell their story?

A. Patients often reveal critical emotional and clinical details through narrative.

B. Storytelling weakens professionalism.

C. Patients dislike being heard fully.

D. Narratives replace diagnosis completely.

84. What is active listening?

A. Fully focusing on and responding thoughtfully to the patient.

B. Listening only for symptoms.

C. Avoiding emotional conversations.

D. Interrupting quickly to improve efficiency.

85. How can listening reveal hidden concerns?

A. Patients often disclose deeper fears when they feel safe and heard.

B. Listening prevents emotional disclosure.

C. Hidden concerns are medically irrelevant.

D. Listening eliminates anxiety permanently.

86. Why does reflective listening improve communication?

A. It confirms understanding and emotional awareness.

B. It weakens trust.

C. It replaces treatment plans.

D. It prevents emotional discussions.

87. How does listening demonstrate respect?

A. Patients feel valued when providers give full attention.

B. Listening weakens authority.

C. Respect only comes from technical skill.

D. Listening prevents efficiency.

88. Why do patients interpret listening as competence?

A. Careful listening suggests thoroughness and attentiveness.

B. Listening replaces clinical knowledge.

C. Patients dislike attentive communication.

D. Listening prevents difficult conversations.

89. What is the impact of divided attention?

A. Patients may feel emotionally unimportant or ignored.

B. Divided attention improves reassurance.

C. Divided attention strengthens trust automatically.

D. Divided attention reduces emotional reactions.

90. Why must providers avoid checklist-only interactions?

A. Patients need human connection, not only task completion.

B. Checklists eliminate empathy automatically.

C. Checklist interactions improve emotional safety completely.

D. Patients prefer emotionally distant communication.

91. How does listening strengthen relationships?

A. Listening builds trust, safety, and emotional connection.

B. Listening weakens professionalism.

C. Listening removes uncertainty permanently.

D. Listening prevents grief.

92. Why do patients share more when they feel heard?

A. Emotional safety increases openness and honesty.

B. Feeling heard weakens trust.

C. Patients prefer emotional distance.

D. Communication becomes unnecessary.

93. How can listening reduce misunderstandings?

A. Clarification improves mutual understanding.

B. Listening increases confusion automatically.

C. Misunderstandings are unrelated to communication.

D. Listening replaces diagnosis.

94. Why is silence sometimes powerful?

A. Silence creates emotional and cognitive processing space.

B. Silence weakens empathy.

C. Silence eliminates communication.

D. Silence prevents honesty.

95. How does listening improve diagnosis?

A. Patients often reveal important clinical clues when fully heard.

B. Listening weakens technical skill.

C. Diagnosis depends only on testing.

D. Listening prevents objectivity.

96. Why must providers listen beyond symptoms?

A. Emotional experiences influence health and coping.

B. Symptoms are emotionally irrelevant.

C. Emotions weaken diagnosis.

D. Listening beyond symptoms reduces professionalism.

97. How can listening improve patient compliance?

A. Patients are more likely to trust providers who truly listen.

B. Listening weakens cooperation.

C. Compliance is unrelated to trust.

D. Listening replaces treatment plans.

98. Why does empathy require listening?

A. Emotional understanding is impossible without hearing the patient fully.

B. Empathy weakens professionalism.

C. Empathy removes the need for communication.

D. Listening prevents emotional awareness.

99. How can providers improve listening habits?

A. By reducing interruptions and remaining fully attentive.

B. By speaking more than the patient.

C. By avoiding emotional topics.

D. By focusing only on documentation.

100. Why is listening foundational to trust?

A. Patients trust providers who make them feel heard and understood.

B. Trust develops independently of communication.

C. Listening weakens authority.

D. Technical skill alone creates trust completely.

Part VI — Difficult Conversations

Questions 101–120

101. Why are difficult conversations emotionally significant?

A. They often involve fear, uncertainty, grief, or vulnerability.

B. Difficult conversations eliminate emotional reactions.

C. Patients rarely remember difficult discussions.

D. Emotions are unrelated to healthcare communication.

102. How should providers deliver bad news?

A. With honesty, compassion, and emotional presence.

B. As quickly as possible without emotion.

C. By avoiding difficult details completely.

D. By focusing only on technical language.

103. Why does pacing matter during difficult discussions?

A. Patients need time to process emotional information.

B. Fast pacing improves emotional comfort automatically.

C. Pacing eliminates sadness.

D. Pacing weakens professionalism.

104. How can providers preserve hope while being honest?

A. By remaining truthful while emphasizing support and next steps.

B. By giving false reassurance.

C. By avoiding difficult realities.

D. By minimizing patient concerns.

105. Why should difficult information be explained clearly?

A. Confusion increases emotional distress and uncertainty.

B. Clarity weakens emotional connection.

C. Patients prefer vague explanations.

D. Clear communication removes grief permanently.

106. How does emotional presence help during bad news?

A. Patients feel less alone during vulnerable moments.

B. Emotional presence weakens professionalism.

C. Emotional presence replaces treatment.

D. Emotional presence prevents grief completely.

107. Why should providers avoid rushed explanations?

A. Rushed communication may feel emotionally cold or dismissive.

B. Rushed explanations improve emotional safety.

C. Rushing eliminates anxiety.

D. Patients prefer rapid conversations during grief.

108. How can providers recognize patient overwhelm?

A. By observing emotional, verbal, and nonverbal reactions carefully.

B. Overwhelm has no visible signs.

C. Emotional reactions are medically irrelevant.

D. Overwhelm improves understanding automatically.

109. Why is silence important during emotional moments?

A. Silence creates emotional processing space.

B. Silence weakens empathy.

C. Silence prevents communication completely.

D. Silence eliminates grief automatically.

110. How should providers respond to crying patients?

A. With calm compassion, patience, and emotional presence.

B. By ignoring emotional reactions.

C. By changing the subject immediately.

D. By discouraging emotional expression.

111. Why must healthcare providers tolerate discomfort?

A. Difficult emotions are unavoidable in patient care.

B. Discomfort weakens professionalism completely.

C. Emotional conversations should always be avoided.

D. Patients prefer emotional distance.

112. How can compassion improve end-of-life conversations?

A. Compassion helps patients and families feel emotionally supported.

B. Compassion weakens honesty.

C. Compassion removes grief permanently.

D. Compassion replaces medical care entirely.

113. Why is honesty critical during uncertainty?

A. Trust depends on truthful communication.

B. Patients prefer false reassurance.

C. Honesty weakens emotional safety.

D. Honesty prevents empathy.

114. How does trust affect difficult decision-making?

A. Patients are more likely to accept guidance from trusted providers.

B. Trust weakens cooperation.

C. Decision-making is unrelated to trust.

D. Trust prevents emotional reactions.

115. Why should providers avoid false reassurance?

A. False reassurance can damage long-term trust.

B. False reassurance improves emotional stability permanently.

C. Patients prefer inaccurate comfort.

D. False reassurance prevents grief.

116. How can providers support grieving families?

A. Through compassion, patience, honesty, and emotional presence.

B. By avoiding emotional discussions.

C. By focusing only on technical details.

D. By discouraging emotional reactions.

117. Why do patients remember difficult conversations vividly?

A. Emotional experiences create lasting memories.

B. Patients quickly forget emotional interactions.

C. Difficult conversations are emotionally unimportant.

D. Technical language removes emotional memory.

118. How can providers reduce trauma during bad news?

A. By communicating calmly, compassionately, and clearly.

B. By avoiding emotional presence.

C. By rushing conversations.

D. By minimizing patient reactions.

119. Why should communication remain calm and structured?

A. Calm structure creates emotional stability during distress.

B. Structure weakens empathy.

C. Emotional conversations should always be unstructured.

D. Calmness removes grief completely.

120. How can empathy improve emotional outcomes?

A. Patients feel emotionally understood and less isolated.

B. Empathy weakens professionalism.

C. Empathy prevents sadness completely.

D. Emotional outcomes are unrelated to empathy.

Part VII — Burnout and Professionalism

Questions 121–140

121. How can burnout affect communication?

A. Burnout may reduce patience, empathy, and emotional presence.

B. Burnout improves emotional connection automatically.

C. Burnout strengthens attentiveness.

D. Burnout eliminates stress completely.

122. Why does exhaustion become visible to patients?

A. Emotional fatigue affects tone, body language, and attentiveness.

B. Exhaustion improves reassurance.

C. Patients cannot recognize emotional fatigue.

D. Exhaustion strengthens communication skills.

123. How can rushed care feel careless?

A. Patients may interpret rushing as emotional disinterest.

B. Rushed care improves emotional safety.

C. Rushing strengthens empathy.

D. Patients prefer emotionally distant communication.

124. Why must providers maintain professionalism under stress?

A. Patients depend on emotional steadiness during vulnerable moments.

B. Stress eliminates the need for professionalism.

C. Professionalism weakens empathy.

D. Emotional reactions improve trust automatically.

125. How can burnout weaken empathy?

A. Emotional exhaustion can reduce emotional availability.

B. Burnout strengthens compassion automatically.

C. Burnout improves patience.

D. Burnout eliminates emotional reactions.

126. Why is self-awareness important in healthcare?

A. Providers must recognize how their emotions affect interactions.

B. Self-awareness weakens professionalism.

C. Emotions are unrelated to patient care.

D. Self-awareness prevents communication.

127. How can providers maintain humanity in high-pressure systems?

A. By remaining intentional, compassionate, and emotionally present.

B. By avoiding emotional connection completely.

C. By focusing only on efficiency.

D. By minimizing patient emotions.

128. Why must providers recognize emotional fatigue?

A. Emotional fatigue can affect communication and patient trust.

B. Fatigue improves emotional awareness automatically.

C. Emotional fatigue strengthens leadership.

D. Fatigue eliminates burnout risk.

129. How can self-care improve patient care?

A. Emotionally healthy providers communicate more effectively.

B. Self-care weakens professionalism.

C. Self-care replaces clinical skill.

D. Self-care eliminates difficult conversations.

130. Why is emotional resilience important?

A. Providers regularly face emotionally difficult situations.

B. Emotional resilience weakens empathy.

C. Resilience prevents sadness completely.

D. Emotional resilience removes stress permanently.

131. How does burnout affect patient trust?

A. Emotional exhaustion may weaken attentiveness and connection.

B. Burnout strengthens emotional safety automatically.

C. Patients ignore provider stress completely.

D. Burnout improves communication.

132. Why should healthcare systems value communication?

A. Communication strongly influences patient experience and outcomes.

B. Communication is unrelated to healthcare quality.

C. Technical skill replaces communication entirely.

D. Patients prefer emotionally distant care.

133. How can efficiency conflict with connection?

A. Excessive focus on speed may weaken emotional presence.

B. Efficiency always improves empathy.

C. Connection weakens professionalism.

D. Patients dislike attentiveness.

134. Why is emotional regulation important for providers?

A. Providers influence the emotional tone of patient encounters.

B. Emotional regulation prevents empathy.

C. Emotional reactions improve communication automatically.

D. Emotional regulation weakens trust.

135. How can providers recover after difficult encounters?

A. Through reflection, support, and emotional self-care.

B. By ignoring emotional stress completely.

C. By avoiding future emotional conversations.

D. By becoming emotionally detached.

136. Why is reflection important in medicine?

A. Reflection improves self-awareness and professional growth.

B. Reflection weakens confidence.

C. Reflection prevents empathy.

D. Reflection removes emotional awareness.

137. How can stress influence tone and behavior?

A. Stress may increase impatience or emotional reactivity.

B. Stress improves communication automatically.

C. Stress eliminates emotional responses.

D. Stress strengthens empathy permanently.

138. Why should providers remain intentional under pressure?

A. Intentional communication preserves emotional connection and trust.

B. Pressure removes the need for empathy.

C. Intentional behavior weakens efficiency.

D. Patients prefer rushed interactions.

139. How does emotional exhaustion affect patient experiences?

A. Patients may feel less emotionally supported or heard.

B. Emotional exhaustion improves reassurance.

C. Patients ignore emotional tone.

D. Emotional exhaustion strengthens compassion.

140. Why must providers protect their own wellbeing?

A. Healthy providers are better able to care for patients effectively.

B. Provider wellbeing is unrelated to patient care.

C. Burnout improves professionalism.

D. Emotional exhaustion strengthens communication.

Part VIII — Leadership and Trust

Questions 141–160

141. Why do patients seek leadership during uncertainty?

A. Leadership provides emotional stability and direction.

B. Leadership removes all fear permanently.

C. Leadership replaces empathy completely.

D. Leadership prevents difficult conversations.

142. What defines effective leadership in medicine

A. Calm guidance, clarity, and emotional steadiness.

B. Emotional detachment and authority only.

C. Avoidance of difficult emotions.

D. Fast decision-making without explanation.

143. Why is direction important during fear?

A. Patients feel safer when they understand what comes next.

B. Direction weakens emotional safety.

C. Fear eliminates the need for guidance.

D. Direction replaces honesty.

144. How can providers create emotional stability?

A. Through calm communication and compassionate leadership.

B. By avoiding emotional discussions completely.

C. By minimizing patient concerns.

D. By focusing only on technical details.

145. Why does clarity strengthen leadership?

A. Clear explanations reduce confusion and uncertainty.

B. Clarity weakens professionalism.

C. Patients prefer vague communication.

D. Confusion improves trust automatically.

146. How can providers inspire confidence?

A. Through calm, honest, and organized communication.

B. By avoiding emotional connection.

C. By speaking aggressively.

D. By minimizing patient questions.

147. Why should leadership remain calm rather than dominant?

A. Calm leadership creates emotional safety and trust.

B. Dominance improves emotional connection automatically.

C. Patients prefer intimidation during vulnerability.

D. Calmness weakens authority.

148. How does trust influence treatment adherence?

A. Patients are more likely to follow guidance from trusted providers.

B. Trust weakens cooperation.

C. Adherence is unrelated to relationships.

D. Trust eliminates uncertainty completely.

149. Why must providers communicate plans clearly?

A. Clear plans help patients feel guided and informed.

B. Plans weaken emotional reassurance.

C. Patients dislike detailed explanations.

D. Communication increases confusion automatically.

150. How can leadership reduce anxiety?

A. Leadership provides structure, clarity, and reassurance.

B. Leadership removes all emotions permanently.

C. Leadership avoids difficult conversations.

D. Leadership weakens trust.

151. Why do patients need guidance during complex decisions?

A. Complex situations increase emotional vulnerability and uncertainty.

B. Patients prefer complete emotional independence.

C. Guidance weakens professionalism.

D. Complexity eliminates emotional reactions.

152. How does confidence affect perception?

A. Calm confidence reassures vulnerable patients.

B. Confidence weakens trust automatically.

C. Confidence replaces empathy.

D. Confidence eliminates fear completely.

153. Why must providers remain composed?

A. Emotional steadiness reassures patients during stress.

B. Emotional reactions improve communication automatically.

C. Composure weakens empathy.

D. Patients prefer emotionally reactive providers.

154. How can transparency strengthen trust?

A. Honest communication helps patients feel respected and informed.

B. Transparency weakens leadership.

C. Patients prefer incomplete information.

D. Transparency increases emotional confusion.

155. Why should providers explain the process of care?

A. Understanding the process reduces uncertainty and fear.

B. Explanations weaken professionalism.

C. Patients prefer emotional confusion.

D. Process explanations replace empathy.

156. How can providers create a sense of partnership?

A. By involving patients respectfully in communication and decision-making.

B. By controlling all conversations completely.

C. By discouraging patient questions.

D. By avoiding emotional discussions.

157. Why is consistency important in healthcare relationships?

A. Consistency builds predictability, trust, and emotional safety.

B. Inconsistency improves reassurance.

C. Patients prefer unpredictability.

D. Consistency weakens emotional connection.

158. How can leadership strengthen emotional safety?

A. Calm guidance helps patients feel protected during uncertainty.

B. Leadership weakens empathy automatically.

C. Emotional safety is unrelated to leadership.

D. Leadership prevents emotional expression.

159. Why do patients remember reassuring providers?

A. Emotional reassurance strongly affects patient memory and trust.

B. Reassurance weakens professionalism.

C. Patients ignore emotional experiences.

D. Reassurance replaces treatment plans.

160. How can trust improve outcomes?

A. Trust improves cooperation, communication, and treatment adherence.

B. Trust weakens emotional safety.

C. Outcomes are unrelated to trust.

D. Trust prevents emotional conversations.

Part IX — Relationship-Centered Care

Questions 161–180

161. Why is relationship-centered care essential?

A. Strong relationships improve trust, communication, and patient experience.

B. Relationships weaken professionalism.

C. Technical skill replaces human connection completely.

D. Patients prefer emotionally distant care.

162. How does connection influence healing?

A. Emotional support can improve coping, trust, and cooperation.

B. Connection weakens treatment outcomes.

C. Healing is unrelated to emotional experience.

D. Connection replaces medical care entirely.

163. Why do patients value feeling understood?

A. Feeling understood creates emotional safety and trust.

B. Patients prefer emotional distance.

C. Understanding weakens professionalism.

D. Emotional support is medically irrelevant.

164. How can providers build long-term trust?

A. Through consistency, honesty, empathy, and attentiveness.

B. By avoiding emotional conversations.

C. By focusing only on technical details.

D. By minimizing patient concerns.

165. Why should providers see patients as individuals?

A. Every patient has unique emotional, personal, and medical needs.

B. Personalization weakens efficiency.

C. Patients prefer standardized emotional care.

D. Individuality prevents professionalism.

166. How does personalization improve communication?

A. Patients feel more respected, understood, and connected.

B. Personalization weakens trust.

C. Communication should always remain emotionally distant.

D. Personalization eliminates professional boundaries.

167. Why is dignity important in patient care?

A. Patients deserve respect during vulnerable moments.

B. Dignity weakens authority.

C. Vulnerability removes the need for respect.

D. Dignity is unrelated to healthcare outcomes.

168. How can providers preserve patient autonomy?

A. By involving patients respectfully in decisions about their care.

B. By controlling all decisions completely.

C. By discouraging patient questions.

D. By avoiding emotional discussions.

169. Why is compassion foundational to medicine?

A. Compassion strengthens trust, comfort, and emotional support.

B. Compassion weakens professionalism.

C. Technical skill eliminates the need for compassion.

D. Compassion prevents honesty.

170. How does trust affect patient engagement?

A. Trusted providers often inspire stronger cooperation and openness.

B. Trust weakens communication.

C. Engagement is unrelated to relationships.

D. Trust prevents emotional reactions.

171. Why must healthcare remain human-centered?

A. Patients are people experiencing vulnerability, not just diagnoses.

B. Human-centered care weakens efficiency.

C. Technical skill replaces emotional needs completely.

D. Patients prefer emotionally detached systems.

172. How can providers strengthen therapeutic relationships?

A. Through empathy, listening, consistency, and emotional presence.

B. By avoiding emotional topics.

C. By minimizing patient fears.

D. By focusing only on diagnosis.

173. Why do patients need emotional safety?

A. Emotional safety encourages openness, honesty, and trust.

B. Emotional safety weakens professionalism.

C. Emotional safety prevents objectivity.

D. Emotional safety eliminates difficult conversations.

174. How can providers improve relational awareness?

A. By reflecting on communication habits and emotional interactions.

B. By avoiding self-awareness.

C. By minimizing emotional reactions.

D. By focusing only on efficiency.

175. Why should communication training begin early?

A. Relationship habits develop early in professional identity.

B. Communication is unrelated to healthcare quality.

C. Emotional awareness weakens medical education.

D. Communication prevents professionalism.

176. How does emotional intelligence affect healthcare?

A. Emotional intelligence improves communication, trust, and leadership.

B. Emotional intelligence weakens competence.

C. Emotional intelligence removes difficult emotions completely.

D. Emotional intelligence replaces medical knowledge.

177. Why is relationship-building teachable?

A. Communication and emotional awareness skills can be practiced and improved.

B. Relationship ability is completely fixed at birth.

C. Training weakens emotional connection.

D. Relationships are unrelated to healthcare.

178. How can providers repair damaged interactions?

A. By acknowledging concerns respectfully and rebuilding trust intentionally.

B. By avoiding emotional discussions.

C. By ignoring patient frustration.

D. By minimizing misunderstandings.

179. Why are relationships central to healing?

A. Human connection influences emotional wellbeing, trust, and cooperation.

B. Healing depends only on technology.

C. Relationships weaken treatment outcomes.

D. Emotional support is medically irrelevant.

180. How can healthcare providers become unforgettable to patients?

A. Through compassion, presence, honesty, and emotional connection.

B. By avoiding emotional interactions.

C. By focusing only on efficiency.

D. By minimizing patient vulnerability.

Part X — Personal Reflection and Growth

Questions 181–200

181. What are your greatest communication strengths?

A. Areas where you consistently build trust and clarity.

B. Areas that weaken all patient relationships.

C. Skills unrelated to patient care.

D. Emotional reactions you completely ignore.

182. What are your greatest weaknesses in patient interaction?

A. Areas requiring reflection, awareness, and improvement.

B. Weaknesses that can never improve.

C. Issues unrelated to communication.

D. Emotional strengths only.

183. How comfortable are you with emotional conversations?

A. Comfort develops through practice, empathy, and experience.

B. Emotional conversations should always be avoided.

C. Emotional discussions weaken professionalism.

D. Comfort eliminates patient vulnerability completely.

184. Why is it important to evaluate whether you interrupt patients too quickly?

A. Interruptions may weaken trust and emotional openness.

B. Interruptions improve emotional safety automatically.

C. Interruptions strengthen listening skills.

D. Patients prefer being interrupted frequently.

185. How well do you tolerate uncertainty?

A. Tolerating uncertainty requires emotional steadiness and communication skill.

B. Uncertainty should always be avoided completely.

C. Tolerating uncertainty weakens professionalism.

D. Uncertainty eliminates patient trust automatically.

186. Why is explaining complex information effectively important?

A. Patients need understandable communication to make informed decisions.

B. Complexity improves trust automatically.

C. Patients prefer confusion.

D. Emotional connection removes the need for explanation.

187. Why should providers check frequently for patient understanding?

A. Patients process information differently during stress and vulnerability.

B. Understanding weakens professionalism.

C. Patients always understand immediately.

D. Clarification prevents empathy.

188. Why should providers remain aware of tone and body language?

A. Nonverbal communication strongly influences emotional perception.

B. Tone is unrelated to patient trust.

C. Body language weakens professionalism.

D. Patients ignore emotional signals.

189. Why is emotional safety important for patients?

A. Emotional safety encourages openness, honesty, and trust.

B. Emotional safety weakens communication.

C. Emotional safety prevents professionalism.

D. Emotional safety eliminates uncertainty permanently.

190. Why is stress management important during patient care?

A. Stress affects emotional presence, patience, and communication.

B. Stress improves empathy automatically.

C. Stress has no effect on patient interactions.

D. Stress strengthens emotional awareness completely.

191. Why is being fully present during patient encounters important?

A. Presence strengthens trust, listening, and emotional connection.

B. Presence weakens efficiency.

C. Patients prefer emotionally distant providers.

D. Presence replaces medical competence.

192. How should providers respond to anxious or angry patients?

A. With calmness, empathy, patience, and emotional regulation.

B. With defensiveness and emotional distance.

C. By avoiding emotional reactions completely.

D. By minimizing concerns immediately.

193. Why is confidence important during difficult conversations?

A. Calm confidence reassures emotionally vulnerable patients.

B. Confidence weakens trust automatically.

C. Confidence replaces empathy entirely.

D. Confidence prevents grief permanently.

194. Why should providers prioritize connection as much as competence?

A. Patients experience emotional connection and competence together.

B. Competence eliminates emotional needs completely.

C. Connection weakens professionalism.

D. Technical skill removes vulnerability automatically.

195. How can providers improve their listening skills?

A. By reducing interruptions and practicing full attentiveness.

B. By speaking more than patients.

C. By focusing only on documentation.

D. By avoiding emotional discussions.

196. How can providers strengthen emotional awareness?

A. Through reflection, empathy, and intentional self-awareness.

B. By avoiding emotions completely.

C. By minimizing patient vulnerability.

D. Emotional awareness cannot improve over time.

197. Why is identifying weak areas important for growth?

A. Awareness allows intentional improvement and learning.

B. Weaknesses should always be ignored.

C. Reflection weakens confidence automatically.

D. Growth is unrelated to self-awareness.

198. Why should providers reflect on concepts that challenged their thinking?

A. Reflection deepens understanding and professional development.

B. Challenging ideas weaken professionalism.

C. Reflection prevents empathy.

D. Difficult concepts should always be avoided.

199. Why is making immediate communication improvements valuable?

A. Small changes can significantly improve patient experience and trust.

B. Communication habits cannot change.

C. Improvement weakens efficiency.

D. Patients ignore communication quality.

200. Why should providers continue strengthening relationship-centered skills?

A. Human connection remains essential to healing, trust, and patient care.

B. Technical skill replaces communication entirely.

C. Relationships are unrelated to healthcare outcomes.

D. Emotional awareness weakens medical competence.

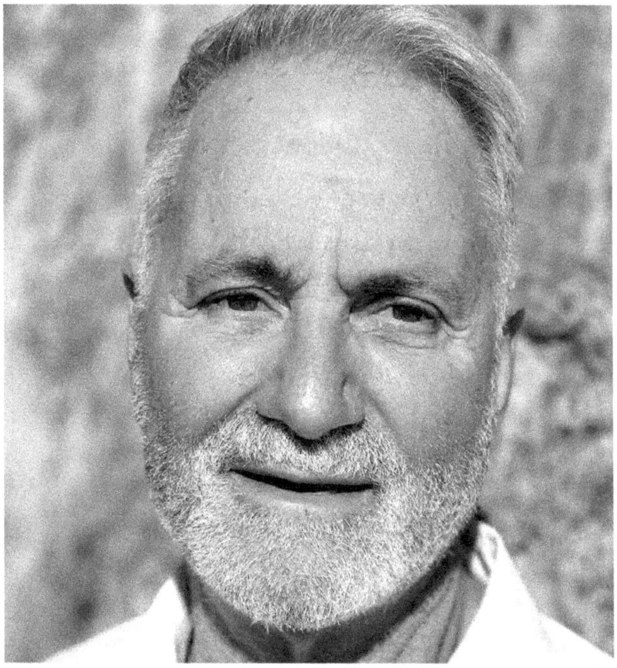

About the Author

Rami Geffner, MD, is an author, educator, healthcare provider, and healthcare advocate recognized for developing a broad body of literary and educational works focused on human behavior, emotional intelligence, communication, and relationship-centered care. A graduate of New Jersey Medical School, where he earned his medical degree.

In addition to his medical career, Dr. Geffner has dedicated much of his professional life to education, writing, and the advancement of human-centered communication within healthcare and personal development. Unlike many contemporary authors who focus on narrow subject areas, he has created an extensive series of educational books, curricula, and learning platforms designed to provide practical, research-informed guidance across emotional, interpersonal, and professional disciplines.

Dr. Geffner is also the founder of the Foundation of Healthy Relationships, Inc., a non-profit organization established to promote healthier interpersonal relationships and emotional awareness. The foundation's educational work began in 2025 with the publication of relationship-centered writings that quickly resonated with readers, earning positive reviews and growing interest. This strong response led to the expansion of a broader educational series focused on modern relationships, emotional development, communication, and the challenges individuals and families face in today's world.

His programs, books, workshops, and educational platforms are designed not only to inform but to provide interactive and practical resources that encourage self-awareness, guided reflection, emotional growth, and real-world application. His work has been recognized for translating complex psychological, behavioral, and relational concepts into accessible guidance for both professionals and the general public.

Among his notable works is his book on dementia, which explores the emotional, relational, and caregiving challenges associated with cognitive decline and patient care. His interviews and educational discussions on podcasts and media platforms have further expanded awareness of relationship-centered communication and emotional wellbeing.

In *Beyond Diagnosis: How to Develop Strong Relationships Between Healthcare Providers and Their Patients*, Dr. Geffner combines decades of medical, clinical, and interpersonal experience to emphasize the critical importance of communication, empathy, trust, compassion, and human connection in healthcare. His insights are intended to benefit healthcare providers, healthcare students, healthcare provider assistants, nurse practitioners, nurses, medical aides, caregivers, and others throughout the healthcare profession who seek to strengthen patient relationships while improving the quality, dignity, and humanity of care.